What *are* you eating?

Distinguish good fat from bad fat in your everyday diet . . . and make healthy alternative choices.

- Love strawberry milkshakes? Cut out the harmful fat with a strawberry-banana breakfast smoothie.
- Addicted to French fries? Satisfy your craving with tasty roasted herb potatoes.
- 2% milk rather than half-and-half or cream can make that wake-up cup of coffee a less unhealthy habit.
- A confirmed carnivore? Organic meats have fewer saturated fats than non-organic cuts, and can help your heart stay healthy.

You'll find many more helpful tips and essential nutritional information in

THE COMPLETE GOOD FAT/BAD FAT, CARB & CALORIE COUNTER

Books by Lynn Sonberg

THE COMPLETE GOOD FAT/BAD FAT, CARB & CALORIE COUNTER

FOODS THAT COMBAT HEART DISEASE

FOODS THAT COMBAT CANCER

THE COMPLETE NUTRITION COUNTER

THE HEALTH NUTRIENT BIBLE: THE COMPLETE ENCYCLOPEDIA OF FOOD AS MEDICINE

THE QUICK AND EASY CHOLESTEROL AND CALORIE COUNTER

THE COMPLETE NUTRITION COUNTER FOR MENOPAUSE

THE FOOD BOOK

ATTENTION: ORGANIZATIONS AND CORPORATIONS
Most Harper paperbacks are available at special quantity discounts for bulk purchases for sales promotions, premiums, or fund raising. For information, please call or write:

Special Markets Department, HarperCollins Publishers, 10 East 53rd Street, New York, New York 10022-5299. Telephone: (212) 207-7528. Fax: (212) 207-7222.

THE COMPLETE GOOD FAT BAD FAT CARB & CALORIE COUNTER

LYNN SONBERG

A Lynn Sonberg Book

HARPER

An Imprint of HarperCollins*Publishers*

This book contains advice and information relating to health care. It is not intended to replace medical advice and should be used to supplement rather than replace regular care by your doctor. It is recommended that you seek your physician's advice before embarking on any medical program or treatment. All efforts have been made to assure the accuracy of the information contained in this book as of the date of publication. The publisher and the author disclaim liability for any medical outcomes that may occur as a result of applying the methods suggested in this book.

HARPER

An Imprint of HarperCollins*Publishers*
10 East 53rd Street
New York, New York 10022-5299

Copyright © 2007 by Lynn Sonberg Book Associates
ISBN: 978-0-06-123127-8
ISBN-10: 0-06-123127-4

All rights reserved. No part of this book may be used or reproduced in any manner whatsoever without written permission, except in the case of brief quotations embodied in critical articles and reviews. For information address Harper paperbacks, an Imprint of HarperCollins Publishers.

First Harper paperback printing: May 2007

HarperCollins® and Harper® are registered trademarks of HarperCollins Publishers.

Printed in the United States of America

Visit Harper paperbacks on the World Wide Web at
www.harpercollins.com

10 9 8 7 6 5 4 3 2 1

If you purchased this book without a cover, you should be aware that this book is stolen property. It was reported as "unsold and destroyed" to the publisher, and neither the author nor the publisher has received any payment for this "stripped book."

CONTENTS

ACKNOWLEDGMENTS

Special thanks are due to Deborah Mitchell for her invaluable help and advice in researching and writing this book.

THE COMPLETE GOOD FAT BAD FAT CARB & CALORIE COUNTER

The Complete Good Fat / Bad Fat, Carb, & Calorie Counter

Good health and good nutrition go hand-in-hand, and so anything that promotes one, promotes and supports the other. The trouble is, books, magazines, TV, and radio are constantly giving people information about what to eat, what not to eat, when to eat it, how much to eat, and how to eat it. To make matters worse, there are many different theories on diet—high-carb, low-carb, low-fat, no-fat, high-fat, count calories, don't count calories; eat according to blood type or the color of your food—the list goes on and on. There are literally hundreds of diets from which to choose, and it's enough to make you throw up your hands and raid the refrigerator.

Not quite so fast. Since you picked up this book, you're concerned about your health and how to choose foods that are nutritious and satisfying. You've made a sound choice, because this book contains concise, relevant nutritional information that can help you shop and eat wisely, regardless of which dietary approach or theory you wish to follow. And here's how to do it.

How This Book Can Help You

If you are like most people, three areas concern you when you think about your health:

1. weight (i.e., losing and/or maintaining a healthy weight);
2. disease prevention (who doesn't want to avoid diabetes, heart disease, or cancer?)
3. overall vitality and sense of well-being.

We have decided to focus this nutrition counter on three important topics: calories, fats (good and bad), and carbohydrates, all of which play essential roles if you want to lose or maintain weight, prevent disease, and maintain general good health—again, *regardless of the diet or nutritional approach you wish to follow.*

Yes, of course it's true that literally scores of nutrients interact with systems in the body to keep you healthy. But the good news is that you really don't need to pay attention to them all. Therefore, in this book we have compiled the latest information on five key factors—calorie content, percentage of calories from fat, total fat, total bad fat, and net carbohydrates, as well as good fat, each explained below—for more than four thousand basic, brand-name, and fast foods that you purchase regularly in supermarkets and fast-food restaurants. Whether your main goal is to prevent or fight disease, to lose weight, or to adopt a more nutritious overall diet for you and your loved ones, *The Complete Good Fat/Bad Fat, Carb, & Calorie Counter* is the only reference guide you'll need. Bring it along whenever you shop or stop at a fast-food establishment, and you'll have the important information you need to make healthy food choices. (Make sure you also look at the "How To Eat For Your Health" section later in this chapter!)

Before you explore the food counter, take the time to read the entire introduction for more detailed information on how the foods we eat impact our health. But first let's take a quick look at each of the categories included in the counter.

- **Calories.** A calorie is the amount of energy needed to raise the temperature of 1 gram of water 1 degree Celsius (or 1.8 degrees Fahrenheit). The number of calories in a food item is the amount of potential energy in that food that your body can "burn" (metabolize) so it can function. Calories are important if you are counting them to help you lose weight, or if you want to prevent disease or enhance overall health, as being overweight is a risk factor for many serious diseases, including cancer, heart disease, gallbladder disease, and diabetes.

- **Percent calories from fat.** The exact percentage of calories people should get from dietary fat remains an area of debate: recommendations range from about 15 to 35 percent, with most experts saying 20 to less than 30 percent is optimal. If you are monitoring your fat intake because you want to lose weight, or because you are concerned about the connection between fat intake and diabetes, heart disease, gallbladder disease, and cancer, then the "percent calories from fat" category will be helpful to you. A more detailed discussion of percent calories from fat can be found later under the heading "How Much Fat Do You Need?"

- **Total fat.** The category "total fat" (in grams) is the sum of saturated, polyunsaturated, monounsaturated, and trans fats, values that are helpful if you are counting fat grams. Based on the percent of calories from fat that you want to consume according to your goal, you can calculate the optimal daily total fat value for you. The handy chart below can help you make that determination.

- **Good fat.** Fats in this category include monounsaturated fats and omega-3 fatty acids. Since we can't tell you the exact number of grams of good fat in any given food (nutrition labels do not provide this information), we did not create a separate category for good fats. However, we did print in boldface the foods that are especially good sources of these good fats, because eating more good fats is just as important as avoiding bad fats.

- **Bad fat.** The category "bad fat" includes the sum of saturated fat and trans fat for each food item. Experts generally recommend that everyone limit intake of bad fat to 10 percent or less of total calories consumed. If you are overweight or have diabetes, heart disease, high blood pressure, cancer, gallbladder disease, or have had a stroke, or you want to help prevent these and other serious diseases, information about the amount of bad fat in your food can help you make healthier choices.

- **Net carbohydrates.** "Net carbs" refers to the total number of carbohydrates minus fiber, glycerin, and sugar alcohols. The reason we provide net carb values instead of total carbs is that these three elements do not have a significant impact on glucose and insulin levels. How do glucose and insulin levels relate to weight loss and diabetes? Basically, carbohydrates raise blood sugar levels, which causes insulin production to increase. The increased insulin pushes sugar into the cells and hinders fat metabolism, making it more difficult to lose weight. Most people who keep track of carbohydrates do so as part of a low-carb weight-loss regimen because they adhere to the concept that eating fewer carbohydrates will lower their glucose and insulin levels, resulting in weight loss. This approach may also help those who are at risk for or who have diabetes.

Calories: Are You Counting?

People often talk about calories—counting calories, burning calories, cutting calories—and their discussion is usually associated with dieting and losing weight. There are many different types of diets, and not all of them emphasize counting calories. However, most experts agree that the bottom line of any diet program is the same, whether you consciously count calories or not: if you eat fewer calories than you burn, you will lose weight; if you eat more calories than you burn, you will gain weight. The types of foods and calories you choose to eat and how you burn those calories (this is where exercise and other factors enter the picture) is up to you.

One important thing to remember if you are counting calories is to look at the serving size of foods. You may find a brand of cookies, for example, that has only 80 calories per serving. That sounds like a good deal if you enjoy cookies, but if you typically eat three or four cookies and the 80 calories refers to one serving (one cookie), your 80-calorie treat may quickly turn into a 300-plus calorie splurge. Therefore, always pay attention to serving sizes, which we have conveniently included in the food counter.

Carbohydrates: Good, Bad, What's The Story?

Not so long ago, carbohydrates were classified as either simple (which includes various sugars such as fructose [fruit sugars], sucrose [table sugar], and glucose), or complex (those composed of three or more sugars bound together). Simple carbs were labeled "bad," while complex ones were "good." But researchers have discovered that carbohydrates are not so simple.

Enter the glycemic index, which measures how quickly and to what degree blood sugar levels increase after you eat carbohydrates. If you eat chocolate or white bread, for example, your blood sugar level will rise sharply and rapidly. These simple-carbohydrate foods have a *high glycemic index*. If, however, you eat brown rice, whole-grain pasta, or broccoli, your blood sugar level will rise much more slowly and moderately. These complex-carbohydrate foods have a low to medium glycemic index, and they can help you maintain even blood sugar levels.

There are several reasons why it is important to maintain even blood glucose and insulin levels. Perhaps the most important one is that it helps reduce the risk of disease, including diabetes, heart disease, stroke, gallbladder disease, and some cancers. Another reason is that widely fluctuating blood glucose levels can make it very difficult to lose weight. If, for example, you eat carbohydrates that cause your blood sugar level to rise rapidly (say, you eat a big chocolate bar), a large amount of glucose enters the bloodstream, causing a "sugar high." The body responds by sending a large amount of insulin into the bloodstream to move the glucose into cells.

Surges in insulin levels, recurring over time, can cause the insulin receptors in the cells to become less sensitive to insulin, resulting in insulin resistance and excess insulin production. This combination can lead to type 2 diabetes or hyperinsulinism (abnormally high levels of insulin in the blood), which can lead to obesity, heart disease, high blood pressure, stroke, and some cancers.

Fiber, which comes in two forms, affects how carbohydrates impact blood sugar levels. Soluble fiber is sticky and is found in oats, fruits, vegetables, dried peas, nuts, seeds, and beans. It binds to glucose (sugar) in the intestinal tract and helps stabilize blood glucose levels. Insoluble fiber is coarse and promotes regularity. Some sources include whole-grain cereals, carrots, celery, tomatoes, zucchini, couscous, and barley. Fiber binds with bile, which helps reduce blood cholesterol levels. Because the bile is excreted with the fiber, the body must manufacture more bile for digestion. It uses cholesterol for this purpose. High-fiber carbohydrates aid weight loss because they increase the bulk of your meal, which in turn helps you feel fuller and less likely to overeat.

Another factor is the acid and fat content of food. The carbohydrates in foods that are higher in fat or acid are metabolized more slowly than foods with lower fat or acid. This is why some foods that contain complex carbohydrates, such as potatoes, cause blood sugar levels to rise quickly and thus act like a simple carbohydrate, while some foods that contain simple carbohydrates, such as oranges, cause blood sugar levels to increase much more slowly and thus act like complex carbohydrates.

Here's the bottom line.

- All carbohydrates—simple, complex, good, bad—break down (metabolize) into sugar (glucose), which the body uses to produce energy.
- Choose natural, unrefined carbohydrates. That means fresh (organic if possible) fruits and vegetables (not potatoes), dried beans and legumes, whole-grain items

(cereals, pastas, breads) and other whole grains, such as quinoa, bulgur, and pearled barley.

Fats: Friends And Foes

Fats are like people: it's good to know which ones are friendly and which ones could do you harm. While good friends enrich your life, negative people can drain you physically, mentally, and emotionally. A secret to well-being and health is to maximize the benefits provided by good friendships and minimize the effects of negative encounters.

So it is with fats. Each of the four main types of fats (saturated, trans, polyunsaturated, and monounsaturated) can be classified as beneficial (a good fat) or damaging (a bad fat). Once you identify good and bad fats, you can optimize your exposure to the former and minimize your exposure to the latter, thus forming a balanced relationship with them and the other basic food components to promote and maintain good health.

Before we look at good fats and bad fats, there are a few things you should know about dietary fats in general. Although the various fats differ in many ways, they all provide 9 calories per gram, which is more than twice as many as the calories supplied by protein and carbohydrates, at 4 per gram. That's not great news if you are trying to lose weight, improve your overall health, or reduce your risk of heart disease and other conditions associated with eating too much bad fat.

But don't be discouraged. Just like you can't avoid all the negative people in your life, you can't avoid all fats—and you don't want to! You *need* some fat in your diet to maintain good health, and that includes a limited amount of bad fat. Some benefits of eating a *balanced* amount of good and bad fats are as follows.

- Fats help your body to absorb the fat-soluble vitamins A, D, E, and K. These vitamins use fat to carry them through the body.
- Fats maintain your brain. Your brain is 60 percent fat. If you deprive your body and brain of an adequate amount of good dietary fats, you may experience problems with mental processes and emotional stability.
- Fats in your diet make you feel fuller longer, which helps you resist the temptation to have between-meal and late-night snacks.
- Hair, skin, and nails need a certain amount of dietary fat to stay healthy.
- Fats promote gastrointestinal health by helping you avoid constipation, bloating, and other digestive problems.
- Fats help ensure proper functioning of the immune system, which wards off infection, stimulates wound healing, and reduces the risk of cancer.
- Fats promote proper nerve functioning.
- Some fats help prevent bone mineral loss.

Bad Fats

Saturated and trans fats are bad fats. *Saturated fats* are usually solid at room temperature and come primarily from animal sources and some tropical oils, such as palm and coconut, and nuts and seeds. The liver uses saturated fats to manufacture cholesterol (see box on page 11).

Consuming too much saturated fat can elevate blood cholesterol levels, which can lead to heart disease and other serious diseases. That's one reason why many experts recommend you limit saturated fat intake. Most of the saturated fat Americans consume comes from animals reared in commercial farms, where they are fed hormones and antibiotics and exposed to pesticides. The amount of saturated fat in these animals is higher than that found in organically fed, free-roaming animals. Therefore, if meats (especially red meats), poultry, and dairy items are part of your diet, buy certified organic products if possible.

Trans fat is created when an unsaturated fat is bombarded with hydrogen atoms to make it partially saturated (i.e., "partially hydrogenated vegetable oil") and solid. This unnatural process is what makes trans fat so harmful. For example, consumption of trans fat

- doubles the risk of heart attack by increasing the levels of LDL cholesterol, decreasing the levels of HDL cholesterol, and promoting the formation of blood clots, which increases the risk of heart attack and stroke;
- increases triglyceride levels, which increases the risk of developing blood clots;
- increases levels of C-reactive protein, a substance that causes inflammation of the blood vessels and thus increases the risk of heart disease;
- damages cardiac metabolism, which can lead to heart disease;
- harms the immune system, liver function, pregnancy and reproductive function, and insulin response and function (especially a problem for diabetics);
- affects the quality of breast milk;
- may increase the risk of developing cancer. Studies suggest these unnatural fats disrupt the natural cell membranes and allow cancer-causing factors to enter cells and damage the nucleus. At least one study has found an increased risk of colon cancer associated with high consumption of trans fat, while another found a higher concentration of trans fat in the breasts of women who had breast cancer.

Clearly, trans fat should be avoided as much as possible. Trans fat, like saturated fat, is solid at room temperature and is made into margarine and shortening. These products are then used in tens of thousands of processed foods, including baked goods, crackers, fried foods, fast foods, and frozen foods.

Fatty Cousins: Cholesterol and Triglycerides

Cholesterol is a waxy substance that consists of fats and proteins and is present in the body both from food intake and from what is produced by the liver (which manufactures 3,000 to 4,000 mg of cholesterol per day). Like fats, cholesterol can be good or bad, which is determined by the type of molecule (lipoprotein) that it travels on as it is transported through the bloodstream.

Cholesterol that is carried on high-density lipoprotein (HDL) cholesterol transports fat from the cells to the liver, where it is excreted and moved throughout the body to be used for cell metabolism and repairs. HDL can help reduce serum cholesterol levels and is therefore considered "good" cholesterol.

Low-density lipoproteins carry oxidized cholesterol from the liver to the cells, but they do not allow the body to use it. The result is that much of the LDL cholesterol accumulates as plaque deposits on the walls of the arteries, hardens with calcium, and becomes atherosclerosis, which can lead to stroke and heart attack. Thus LDL cholesterol is directly associated with an increased risk of cardiovascular disease and is "bad."

Cholesterol is also "good" when it acts as an antioxidant and protects cells from free radical damage (free radicals are molecules that harm cells) and against atherosclerosis, cancer, and other serious medical conditions. Cholesterol is also critically important for the production of many steroid hormones (e.g., estrogen, testosterone, progesterone, DHEA, pregnenolone) and vitamin D.

The basic component of a fat is the *triglyceride*, which consists of a base substance called glycerol to which are attached three fatty acid chains. When triglycerides are digested (metabolized), they break down into these fatty acids and glycerol and are transported from the intestinal tract into the lymphatic system and finally deposited into the bloodstream.

A diet high in fat, especially bad fats, increases your risk of developing high triglyceride levels. Triglycerides cause the blood to thicken, therefore the greater the amount of triglycerides in the blood, the harder the heart has to work to circulate the blood through your body.

Good Fats

Monounsaturated fat is a good fat and the type that many health-care practitioners encourage their patients to choose over saturated and some polyunsaturated fats (see "Polyunsaturated Fats"). Unlike polyunsaturated fat, which lowers both LDL and HDL cholesterol, monounsaturated fat selectively reduces the more damaging LDL cholesterol while it promotes high levels of HDL, and also reduces triglyceride levels.

Studies show that people who consume olive oil as their main source of fat (olive oil is very high in monounsaturated fat) have the lowest rates of cardiovascular disease in the world. Researchers have also found that the most significant benefit in terms of a reduced risk of cardiovascular disease is seen in people who substitute monounsaturated fats for saturated fats in their diet. Because saturated fats increase the risk of heart disease and monounsaturated fats reduce it, you can maximize your health benefit when you reduce your intake of the bad fat and increase your consumption of the good fat. Foods high in monounsaturated fats include olives, olive oil, peanuts, avocados, and cashews.

Also in the good-fat category are omega-3 fatty acids, a type of polyunsaturated fat found primarily in certain fish and some oils, nuts, and leafy green vegetables. You can read more about the many benefits of omega-3 fatty acids below.

Good and Bad: Polyunsaturated Fats

Many people are confused about polyunsaturated fats: Are they good or bad? The short answer is, yes, they can be both. The longer answer requires that we look at two types of polyunsaturated fats—omega-3 and omega-6 essential fatty acids.

Omega-3 fatty acids provide a long list of benefits.

- Improved brain function.
- Enhanced mood.
- Improved concentration and mental processing.
- Improved energy production.
- Decrease of most risk factors for cardiovascular disease, including high triglycerides, blood pressure, fibrinogen, and platelet stickiness.
- Reduction of cancer risk.
- Help reduce fat production in the body.
- Improved health of the gut and reduced gut inflammation.
- Reduced allergy symptoms.
- Speedier healing from injuries.

- Improved bone mineral retention, which helps inhibit the development of osteoporosis.
- Reduced inflammation. Omega-3 fatty acids convert into a substance called prostaglandin 3, which has anti-inflammatory properties.
- Improved sleep in some people.
- Improved hormone functions.
- Needed for kidney and liver functions.
- Instrumental in pregnancy, sperm formation, and the menstrual cycle.

Unfortunately, most Americans don't consume nearly enough omega-3s and/or they consume an amount that is out of balance with their intake of omega-6 fatty acids (see "Omega-6:Omega-3 Ratio" below).

Omega-6 fatty acids are found mainly in vegetable oils and get a mixed review. Although natural, virgin polyunsaturated oils (e.g., corn, soy, safflower) reduced the risk of cardiovascular disease by 19 percent in some studies, their highly processed counterparts that are so common on today's market shelves have been stripped of most of their healthful properties. A benefit of omega-6 fatty acids is that they are important in blood vessel structure and skin health. They also convert into a substance called prostaglandin 1, which has anti-inflammatory properties.

The downside of polyunsaturated fats is that they produce free radicals when they are heated (as in frying) or when they are metabolized, and these molecules can damage healthy tissue, speed up aging, and harm the immune system. Therefore the best way to reap any benefits from polyunsaturated fats is to use them unheated (as oils) or enjoy them in fish, almonds, and walnuts.

Omega-6:Omega-3 Ratio. Nutritional experts generally

agree that the ratio of omega-6 to omega-3 should favor the former, although not everyone agrees on what that ratio should be. More seem to agree that a ratio of 4-to-1 is best, yet Americans are closer to a 20-to-1 ratio or greater. Therefore, try to reduce your omega-6 intake while increasing omega-3 consumption to close the gap. That means eating fewer fried foods and vegetable oils and consuming more fish rich in omega-3, such as salmon, herring, sardines, and tuna. To help you find foods that contain omega-3, they are in bold-faced type in the food counter.

How Much Fat Do You Need?

Some experts, including the American Heart Association and the National Cancer Institute, recommend you consume no more than 30 percent of your daily caloric intake from fat, although others, including dietary fat expert Udo Erasmus, Ph.D, author of *Fats That Heal, Fats That Kill,* say 15 to 20 percent is ideal. The *Dietary Guidelines for Americans 2005*, issued by the U.S. Department of Health and Human Services, suggests a range of 20 to 35 percent (although the 35 percent is not viewed favorably by many experts).

In addition to your *total fat* intake, you also need to consider the amount of *bad fats*—saturated plus trans fats—included in that total. Basically, you want to minimize the amount of bad fats to less than 10 percent of calories consumed while you focus on eating *good* fats. (*For your convenience, in the Food Counter we have in bold-faced type the foods that contain an appreciable amount of good fats.*)

What should your optimum fat intake be? That depends on your current health and goals. You can use the following table to help you make a decision, while also thinking about the following considerations.

- If you want to improve your health but don't want to make major changes in your diet, choose the 30 percent column. If you are overweight, you will probably lose some weight if you follow this suggestion.
- If you want to improve your health and/or lose weight and are willing to make more significant dietary changes, then choose the 25 percent column.
- If you want to lose weight more rapidly and/or you want to increase the health benefits that many experts believe a low-fat diet can provide, then choose the fat gram quota under the 15 or 20 percent column.

Desired	**Maintenance**	**Calories From Fat**			
Weight	**Calories**	**15%**	**20%**	**25%**	**30%**
Women					
100	1,500	25 g	33 g	42 g	50 g
120	1,800	30 g	40 g	50 g	60 g
140	2,100	35 g	47 g	58 g	70 g
160	2,400	40 g	53 g	67 g	80 g
Men					
135	2,025	34 g	45 g	56 g	68 g
155	2,325	39 g	52 g	65 g	78 g
175	2,625	44 g	58 g	73 g	88 g
195	2,925	49 g	65 g	81 g	98 g

You can use this book to determine the amount of fat you are consuming *now,* before you change your fat intake. Record everything you eat for a few days. Once you know where you are *now,* you can better work toward your goal. Now let's look at the different types of fat and their impact on your health.

Fat, Calories, and Disease

Diabetes

About 18 million adults in the United States have type 2 diabetes. This fact certainly is cause for concern, but two more reasons heighten it considerably.

- 41 million Americans have prediabetes, a condition in which blood sugar levels are just shy of those characteristic of full-blown type 2 diabetes.
- Type 2 diabetes, once seen nearly exclusively in adults, is now developing in children and adolescents in alarmingly increasing numbers.

Fortunately, type 2 diabetes is preventable. Excess weight and a poor diet are two of the main factors responsible for 90 percent of the type 2 cases of diabetes in women, according to the results from the Nurses' Health Study. Being overweight, for example, increases your chances of developing type 2 diabetes sevenfold, and the types of fat you eat can affect the development of diabetes. This book can help you prevent diabetes because it identifies foods that contain bad fats, helps you count calories, and identifies foods that are low in fat overall.

Diabetes prevention cannot be emphasized enough, especially since the consequences of having the disease are serious and often deadly. For example, compared with people who don't have diabetes, people with the disease

- have a two to four times higher risk of dying of heart disease;
- have a two to four times higher risk of stroke;
- are at high risk of becoming blind. Diabetes is the leading cause of new cases of blindness among adults.

- are at high risk of end-stage renal disease. Diabetes is the leading cause of this condition.
- have a twofold greater risk of death overall.

Once you balance your fat intake, you'll have a healthier diet and, very likely, a healthier weight, which will reduce your risk of developing diabetes.

Heart Disease

Many factors are involved in the development of heart disease, and a key one is the amount of bad fat in the diet. This fact was made clear in a statement made by Jacques Rossouw, MD, project officer for the Women's Health Initiative, which studied the data from more than 48,000 women. In a February 2006 news release by the National Institutes of Health, Dr. Rossouw noted that "just reducing total fat intake does not go far enough to have an impact on heart disease risk." Rather, he emphasized that he and his colleagues "saw trends towards greater reductions in cholesterol and heart disease risk in women eating less saturated and trans fat." While the U.S. Dietary Guidelines for Americans recommends that adults keep saturated fats to less than 10 percent of calories, and that most of the fats consumed come from monounsaturated and polyunsaturated fats, people with heart disease or who are at high risk for the disease should strive for 5 or 6 percent saturated fats.

Some experts estimate that 30,000 premature coronary heart disease deaths per year can be attributed to consumption of trans fats, while others place the number at 100,000. Regardless of the exact number, the point is that these deaths, or most of them, could be avoided by making dietary changes. Reducing consumption of bad fat is a major step in reducing your risk of heart disease.

Cancer

What does fat have to do with cancer? Being overweight or obese is associated with a higher risk of colon, breast, and prostate cancers, while being physically active can reduce your cancer risks. In fact, the American Cancer Society notes that one third of cancer deaths are related to diet and inactivity.

Although a high-fat diet is not believed to directly cause cancer, it seems to promote cancer development in people who are exposed to cancer-causing agents (carcinogens). Therefore, a high-fat diet can cause the body to secrete a greater amount of certain hormones, such as estrogen, that are associated with certain types of cancer, such as breast cancer. A high-fat diet may also alter the characteristics of cells, making them more vulnerable to carcinogens. High-fat diets are also typically high in cholesterol, and when cholesterol breaks down in the colon, some of the by-products act like estrogen and other female hormones, which can stimulate breast tissue and cause tumors.

High-fat diets also predispose people to colorectal cancer. It appears that the breakdown of fat in the colon produces carcinogens. Because fat moves more slowly through the lower intestine than do carbohydrates or protein, the fats and the harmful byproducts have more time to cause damage. A high-fiber diet may help rid the bowel of carcinogens and help reduce the risk of cancer.

How To Eat For Your Health

Above all, the foundation of a nutritious, health-promoting diet includes lots of fresh fruits and vegetables, whole grains and cereals, legumes, nuts and seeds, certain cold-water fatty fish, healthy oils (e.g., olive, flax), eggs and low-fat dairy, and/or lean animal protein. (All foods should be organic and/or free-range when possible.) That being said, you can choose the foods to achieve such a diet with help from the food counter and other information in this book.

Toward that goal, in this section we offer some practical tips on how to increase fiber and good carbohydrate intake, reduce bad fats and substitute healthier ones, and reduce fat intake overall.

Up with Fiber in Your Diet

Once you reduce bad fat intake, you will likely notice an increase in your intake of high-fiber, good carbohydrate foods. This is a natural, healthy shift, and here's why.

Fiber is a noncaloric, indigestible plant material that makes you feel full and also helps keep your intestinal tract healthy by assisting in the elimination of waste. High-fiber foods such as whole-grain breads and cereals, legumes, and fruits and vegetables generally take longer to eat than high-fat foods, which gives your stomach the 20 minutes or so it needs to send a message to the brain that it is full. The result is that you tend to eat less.

Tips on Healthy Eating

Regardless of the dietary approach you choose, the following tips can help you and your family eat a more nutritious diet that contains less bad fat and less total fat, and to make more informed choices when it comes to calories and carbohydrates. Many of these tips offer more than one benefit; that is, they reduce bad fat, reduce calories, and provide better quality carbohydrates.

- Opt for nonfat or low-fat dairy foods rather than full-fat items in recipes unless it specifically states that the quality will be affected.
- Use 2 percent milk instead of half-and-half, cream, or powdered coffee creamers for your coffee.
- Substitute butter with a spread that contains olive oil, available in the margarine section of the grocery.
- Use olive oil, balsamic vinegar, herbs, or salsa on salads instead of ranch or other creamy dressings.
- Use olive oil for cooking.
- Use two egg whites instead of one whole egg and three egg whites instead of two eggs. This allows you to nearly eliminate cholesterol and fat.
- When greasing a pan or cookie sheet, use vegetable oil spray rather than liquid oil.
- When a recipe calls for milk, you may be able to use broth or fruit juice, depending on the type of dish you are making. When making mashed potatoes, for example, use vegetable broth or nonfat chicken broth instead of milk. The potatoes will have less fat and more flavor.
- Rather than using cream to thicken gravies and soups, add pureed cooked vegetables, farina, or bread crumbs.
- Add one or more plant-based meals to your menu plans each week. Plant-based dishes are typically low in fat, have no cholesterol (if they are egg and/or dairy free), and lower in calories than animal-based dishes. You can substitute low-fat vegetarian "meats" for animal products in recipes such as lasagna, chili, stews, and casseroles.
- When making meat or poultry, use a steamer rack, which allows fat to drip away from the food.
- Flavor your cooked vegetables with low-fat salsa, lemon juice, or a few drops of olive oil or chili oil instead of butter or margarine.

- Remove excess fat from meat and skin from poultry before you cook it.
- Use low-fat yogurt on your baked potatoes instead of sour cream.
- Read labels. Avoid foods that have the following words in the ingredient list: hydrogenated or partially hydrogenated oil, oil, shortening, lard.
- When stir-frying, use broth and just a few drops of oil.
- Avoid processed meats such as hot dogs, pepperoni, and cold cuts. Instead, choose unprocessed cold cuts such as roast beef, baked ham, and turkey breast. These options also contain less sodium.
- Prepare fresh vegetables instead of using frozen, prepared vegetable products, such as broccoli with cheese sauce or beans in butter sauce.
- Prepare a list of low-fat dishes that you and your family enjoy and keep the ingredients on hand for them so you'll always be ready to make them.
- To make sure you always have low-fat ingredients on hand, prepare a standard shopping list with "must have on hand" items, such as whole-grain cereals and pasta, low-fat cheese, olive oil, salsa, fresh vegetables, fresh fruits, vegetable broth, skinless poultry, fresh fish, your favorite herbs, brown rice, beans, and low-fat yogurt.
- When cooking meat and poultry, prepare them a day ahead, refrigerate them, and skim off the hardened fat before you reheat.
- Enjoy pasta without fattening sauces. Use salsa, a few drops of olive oil, minced garlic, and pureed cooked vegetables instead.
- Prepare your own microwavable meals instead of buying low-calorie frozen entrees or dinners that are often high in fat. Precook the food of your choice (e.g., chicken,

fish, lean beef, rice, vegetables) and place them in reusable microwavable containers, then freeze. When it is time to reheat them, add about a tablespoon of defatted broth to the container to restore moistness.

- Use beans, vegetables, or whole grains to replace some of the meat content of meatloaf or burgers.
- Coat chicken and fish in breadcrumbs instead of batter and bake them instead of frying them.
- Oven-fry potatoes instead of making or buying French fries.
- Choose turkey or chicken sausages instead of beef or pork sausages.

Two-Day Menu and Recipes

Day 1

BREAKFAST

Breakfast Smoothie
½ whole-wheat bagel with all-natural fruit jelly
6 oz orange juice (optional)
Hot herbal or green tea

LUNCH

Tuna Pasta Lunch Salad
Handful of macadamia nuts
Tea

DINNER

Chicken and Pears
Curried Rice
Festive Mango Slaw
Tea

Day 2

BREAKFAST

Pumpkin Oatmeal
6 oz orange or pineapple juice
Hot tea or coffee

LUNCH

Gazpacho
Nutty Rhubarb Muffin
Seltzer with lemon

DINNER

Zesty Fish Fillets
Sweet and Sour Vegetables
Roasted Herbed Potatoes
Hot tea or coffee

Recipes

BREAKFAST SMOOTHIE

Two 8-oz servings; per serving: 100 calories, 1g fat, 21g carbohydrates

¾ cup strawberries, remove stems
¼ cup pineapple chunks
4 oz vanilla low-fat yogurt
¼ cup orange or pineapple juice
6–10 ice cubes

Place all ingredients in a blender except ice cubes and blend till smooth, then add ice cubes and blend until smooth again.

TUNA PASTA LUNCH SALAD

Serves 4; per serving: 240 calories, 8g fat, 23g carbohydrates

1½ cups elbow pasta (whole wheat)
1 12-oz can water-packed tuna, drained
4 scallions, chopped
12 cherry tomatoes
¼ cup black olives, chopped
3 Tbs balsamic vinegar
1½ Tbs olive oil
2 garlic cloves, crushed
1 tsp Dijon mustard
6 cups mixed salad greens

Prepare the pasta according to package directions, drain, and rinse with cold water. Place cooled pasta in a large bowl and add the tuna, scallions, tomatoes, and olives. In another bowl, whisk together the oil, vinegar, mustard, and garlic. Pour the dressing over the pasta mixture and toss to coat. Spoon the tuna pasta mixture over the salad mix and serve.

CHICKEN AND PEARS

Serves 4; per serving: 250 calories, 5.5g fat, 27g carbohydrates

5 cups peeled pears, chopped (about 1½ to 2 lbs)
8 chicken thighs, skinned
4 cloves garlic, chopped
½ tsp ground cinnamon
½ tsp salt
¼ tsp black pepper

Preheat oven to 475 F. Combine the pears, cinnamon, and garlic in a large bowl. Add the salt and stir well. Spray oil into the bottom of a baking pan and spread the pear mixture on the bottom of the pan. Arrange the chicken on top of the pear mixture and sprinkle with salt and pepper. Bake for 25 minutes or until the chicken is cooked through.

CURRIED RICE

Serves 8; per serving: 196 calories, 3g fat, 31g carbohydrates

2 tsp olive oil
1 cup bell pepper, diced
½ cup sliced onion
½ cup chopped celery
2 Tbs curry powder
3 cups hot cooked rice
2 Tbs lime juice
½ tsp salt
1 20-oz can pineapple chunks, drained
1 15-oz can black beans, drained
½ cup cashews

Heat oil in a skillet. Saute the pepper, celery, and onions for 2 to 3 minutes. Add the curry and stir for 30 seconds. Combine the cooked rice, lime juice, and salt in a bowl. Stir in the cooked vegetables, pineapple, and beans. Sprinkle with cashews right before serving. May be served warm or at room temperature.

FESTIVE MANGO SLAW

Serves 6; per serving: 43 calories, 0g fat, 11g carbohydrates

2½ cups shredded cabbage (green and/or red)
1 medium jicama, shredded
1 mango, chopped
2 green onions, chopped
½ cup shredded carrots
2 Tbs lime juice

Combine all ingredients except lime juice in a bowl and mix well. Sprinkle on juice, chill and serve.

PUMPKIN OATMEAL

Serves 4; per serving: 242 calories, 3g fat, 40g carbohydrates

2 cups quick or old-fashioned oats
3 cups fat-free milk
½ cup canned pumpkin
¼ tsp pumpkin pie spice
1 Tbs raisins
⅛ tsp cinnamon
Brown sugar to taste

Bring the milk to a boil in a saucepan. Stir in the oats and cook over medium heat for about 5 minutes. Add the pumpkin, brown sugar, and spices and stir until heated through. Stir in raisins before serving.

GAZPACHO

Serves 6; per serving: 62 calories, 2g fat, 9g carbohydrates

3 cups tomato juice
1 cup chopped tomatoes (peeled)
1 cup chopped cucumber (peeled)
1 cup green pepper, chopped
½ cup green onion, chopped
2 Tbs red wine vinegar
1 Tbs olive oil
1 clove garlic, minced
4 or more drops Tabasco sauce, to taste
Salt and pepper to taste

Blend all ingredients together except salt, pepper, and Tabasco sauce. Taste, then add seasonings as desired. Chill before serving.

NUTTY RHUBARB MUFFINS

Makes 8; per serving: 81 calories, 7g fat, 27g carbohydrates

½ cup whole-wheat flour
¼ cup sugar
1 Tbs baking powder
½ tsp ground cinnamon
½ cup nonfat milk
1 egg, beaten
2 Tbs canola oil
1 cup chopped rhubarb, fresh or frozen (thawed)
¼ cup chopped walnuts or pecans

Preheat oven to 350 F. Coat an 8-cup muffin pan with nonstick cooking spray or line with paper muffin cups. Combine flour, sugar, baking powder, and cinnamon in a large bowl and mix well. Add rhubarb and nuts. In another bowl, combine milk, egg, and oil. Pour milk mixture into rhubarb mixture and stir until dry ingredients are moistened. Spoon batter into muffin pan. Bake for 20–25 minutes.

ZESTY FISH FILLETS

Serves 4; per serving: 121 calories, 1g fat, 6g carbohydrates

Four 4-oz cod, haddock, or pollock fillets
½ tsp salt, or to taste
1 cup tomato sauce
2 tsp ground cumin
1 tsp ground black pepper
2 Tbs vermouth or white wine
1 tsp dried oregano
Olive oil spray
1 lemon, halved

Preheat oven to 375 F. Lightly spray a baking pan with the olive oil. Season fish with salt and pepper and arrange in the pan. Combine sauce, wine, cumin, and oregano and pour over the fish. Cover the pan with foil and bake for 20 to 25 minutes or until the fillet centers are opaque. Squeeze ½ of the lemon over the fish and cut the other half into 4 wedges to serve with the fish.

SWEET AND SOUR VEGETABLES

Serves 4; per serving: 65 calories, 1g fat, 13g carbohydrates

1 cup broccoli florets
1 cup cauliflower florets
1 cup shredded cabbage
2 medium carrots, sliced
1 large red bell pepper, sliced
¼ cup water
2 tsp cornstarch
1 tsp sugar
⅓ cup unsweetened pineapple juice
1 Tbs reduced-sodium soy sauce
1 Tbs rice vinegar
½ tsp dark sesame oil

Combine all the vegetables in a large nonstick skillet. Add water and bring to a boil. Reduce heat, cover, and steam for 4 minutes. While the vegetables are steaming, combine the cornstarch, sugar, pineapple juice, soy sauce, and vinegar in a small bowl and blend. Drain the vegetables in a colander. Place the soy sauce mixture into the skillet. Return the vegetables to the skillet and toss with the sauce. Add the sesame oil before serving.

ROASTED HERB POTATOES

Serves 4; per serving: 114 calories, 2g fat, 21g carbohydrates

1 lb Idaho or russet potatoes
2 Tbs finely chopped parsley
2 tsp olive oil
½ tsp each: garlic powder, onion powder, dried crushed thyme leaves, ground red pepper (optional)
¼ tsp black pepper

Preheat oven to 400 F. Peel potatoes and cut each one into 8 wedges. Place the remaining ingredients in a bowl and toss with the potatoes until coated. Place the potatoes on an ungreased oven tray and bake for 50 minutes, turning the wedges after about 25 minutes.

SNACKS

Berries: blueberries, strawberries, raspberries
One-quarter avocado with lemon juice
Gelatin dessert with fruit
Hot-air popped corn sprayed with nonfat cooking oil and sprinkled with garlic powder, ground cumin, and/or salt

Eating Out

You can eat out and watch your fat intake at the same time if you plan ahead or go armed with some simple strategies. Here are some tips.

- Avoid menu items that say fried, creamed, or buttered. Instead, look for the words poached, baked, steamed, roasted, or braised.
- If you are not on a strictly low-fat regimen, items lightly browned or sauteed in olive oil—a good fat—are acceptable.

- Even if the menu says an item is low-fat, it may come swimming in cream sauce. Always ask the waitperson for the ingredients and how an item is served. If he or she doesn't know, ask that they check with the chef. If it comes with a sauce, ask for a small amount on the side or refuse it.
- When ordering a salad, always ask for the dressing on the side. If olive oil and vinegar are not offered as an option, request them.
- Dine at restaurants that offer heart-healthy or low-fat entrees.
- Substitute a salad or baked potato for french fries, coleslaw, or other high-fat side dishes. If you are on a low-carb diet, ask for a vegetable instead of the baked potato.
- If you are watching your carbs, avoid the bread basket, especially before your meal. If you want to have bread with your meal, choose whole-grain varieties, which will have less impact on blood sugar, and eat a moderate portion.
- Ask your server whether the restaurant offers low-carb entrees and ask to see the carbohydrate values for the items.
- To order a low-carb burger or other sandwich, ask for the item without the bun or bread, or for only one slice or half a bun (and that slice or half should be whole grain).
- Control serving sizes by asking for a side-dish or appetizer-size serving or by bringing part of your meal home with you.
- When ordering pizza, ask for vegetable toppings and little or no cheese.
- At fast-food restaurants, choose the salads (watch out for the dressing!) or grilled sandwiches.

- Bring this book with you whenever you eat out, especially at fast-food restaurants.

Serving Sizes

Many people underestimate the amount of food they eat while overestimating the recommended portion sizes for many foods. To help you determine standardized portion sizes, here are a few clues.

- A baseball: a serving of fruit or vegetables is about the size of a baseball.
- A deck of cards or your palm (without fingers): this comparison is often given to determine a serving of meat, fish, or poultry.
- Golf ball: one quarter cup of dried fruit or nuts.
- Four dice: equals about 1 ounce of cheese.
- Ping-pong ball: 2 tablespoons of peanut butter, butter, cream cheese, or similar foods.
- Tennis ball: about one-half cup of ice cream.
- Compact disc: one serving of pancake or a small waffle.
- Rounded handful: about one-half cup cooked or raw vegetables or one-half cup cooked pasta or rice.

According to the U.S. Department of Agriculture, one serving equals the following.

- 1 slice of whole-grain bread
- ½ bagel
- ½ cup cooked pasta, rice, or mashed potatoes
- 1 small pancake
- 2 medium cookies
- ½ cup cooked or raw vegetables

- 1 small baked potato
- ½ grapefruit or mango
- ½ cup berries
- 1 medium apple
- ¾ cup vegetable juice
- 1cup milk or yogurt
- 1 chicken breast
- 1½ ounces of cheddar cheese
- ¼ lb hamburger patty

On Your Way

Whether you want to lose weight or maintain it; if you have diabetes or are trying to prevent it; or if you've decided to adopt a healthier lifestyle to prevent disease, this book can help you. *The Complete Good Fat/Bad Fat, Carb, & Calorie Counter* provides you with vital information on more than four thousand foods so you can make healthier food choices at home and away. As always, you should consult your physician before you make any major changes in your diet.

FOOD CHARTS

How to Read the Charts

ABBREVIATIONS AND SYMBOLS USED

dia = diameter
f-f = fat-free
g = gram
n/a = not available
oz = ounce
pc(s) = piece(s)

pkg = package (refers to a complete frozen meal, entrée, or other item that is considered to be one serving as packaged)
Tbs = tablespoon
tsp = teaspoon
< = less than

Total Fat = the sum total of saturated, trans, polyunsaturated (which includes omega-3 fatty acids), and monounsaturated fats, in grams. **Bad Fats** = the sum total of saturated and trans fats, in grams. **Net Carbs** = total carbohydrates minus fiber, in grams. **NOTE:** Products **in bold-face** type contain an appreciable amount of good fats—monounsaturated and/or omega-3 fatty acids.

Nutritional information for foods that require the addition of ingredients (e.g., cake mixes, some boxed dinners) may be given for the mix only or for when the item is prepared according to package directions.

Mix = values given are for the mix only, as packaged. For some products, you may substitute ingredients that will have a significant impact on the prepared food's fat and calorie values. For example, if a cake mix requires the addition of milk, margarine, and egg, you have the option to substitute skim milk for whole milk, low-fat spread for margarine, and egg white rather than a whole egg, all of which will reduce the final fat and calorie content.

Prep. = prepared according to package directions.

Product and Portion Size	**Calories**	**% Cal from Fat**	**Total Fat (g)**	**Bad Fat (g)**	**Net Carbs (g)**
ACORN SQUASH, boiled, mashed, ½ cup	42	1%	0	0	8
ALMONDS					
Dry roasted, no salt, 1 oz	**169**	**74%**	**15**	**1**	**2**
Oil roasted, no salt, 1 oz	**172**	**76%**	**16**	**1**	**2**
ANCHOVIES, in oil, drained, 1 oz	59	41%	3	1	0
APPLE JUICE					
Eden Foods, organic, 8 oz	90	0%	0	0	24
Martinelli's, 8 oz	140	0%	0	0	35
Minute Maid, frozen, prep., 8 oz	110	0%	0	0	28
Mott's 100%, bottled, 8 oz	120	0%	0	0	29
Mott's Plus Light Juice Beverage, 8 oz	60	0%	0	0	15
Walnut Acres, organic, 8 oz	110	0%	0	0	29
Apple white grape					
Minute Maid, frozen, prep., 1 box	100	0%	0	0	25
APPLESAUCE					
Lucky Leaf Deluxe, cinnamon, ½ cup	100	0%	0	0	23
Mott's original, ½ cup	110	0%	0	0	26
Mott's unsweetened, ½ cup	50	0%	0	0	13

Product and Portion Size	Calories	% Cal from Fat	Total Fat (g)	Bad Fat (g)	Net Carbs (g)
Musselman's, ½ cup	90	0%	0	0	20
APPLES					
Raw, with skin, medium	72	2%	0	0	16
Raw, without skin, medium	61	0%	0	0	14
Dried, sulfured, 1 cup	209	2%	0	0	50
APPLE BUTTER, 1 Tbs	29	0%	0	0	7
APRICOTS, fresh, 1	17	0%	0	0	3
Dried, 1 oz	68	0%	0	0	16
Del Monte, canned, halves, drained ½ cup	100	0%	0	0	25
Del Monte, canned, lite halves, ½ cup	60	0%	0	0	15
S&W, sun apricots, ½ cup	90	0%	0	0	21
S&W, whole, ½ cup	120	0%	0	0	28
APRICOT NECTAR, organic (Santa Cruz) 8 oz	120	0%	0	0	28
ARTICHOKE					
Jerusalem, 1 cup slices	114	0%	0	0	24
Birds Eye, hearts, frozen, 12 pcs	40	9%	1	0	2
ASIAN FOODS (canned, boxed); also see Frozen Dinners					
Taste of Thai, coconut ginger noodles, 1 cup prep.	280	18%	7	7	52

Product and Portion Size	Calories	% Cal from Fat	Total Fat (g)	Bad Fat (g)	Net Carbs (g)
Taste of Thai, red curry noodles, 1 cup prep.	280	21%	8	4	49
Taste of Thai, Pad thai noodles, 1 cup prep.	240	8%	2	0.5	46
Thai Pavilion, Authentic pad thai, ⅓ pkg	230	15%	4	1	44
Thai Pavilion, Garlic basil, ⅓ pkg	220	20%	5	1	40
Thai Pavilion, Peanut satay, ⅓ pkg	210	29%	7	2	31
Thai Pavilion, Thai green curry, ⅓ pkg	170	29%	5	3.5	26
ASPARAGUS, fresh, cooked, no salt, ½ cup	20	0%	0	0	2
Birds Eye, cuts, ¾ cup	20	0%	0	0	3
Birds Eye, spears, 7	20	0%	0	0	3
Birds Eye, stir-fry, 1 cup cooked	80	0%	0	0	13
Del Monte, canned, cuts & tips, ½ cup	20	0%	0	0	2
Del Monte, canned, spears, 7 spears	20	0%	0	0	3
Green Giant, cuts, no sauce, ½ cup cooked	20	0%	0	0	2
Green Giant, canned spears, 5	20	0%	0	0	2
Green Giant, canned spears, low sodium, ½ cup	20	0%	0	0	2
AVOCADO, California, 1	**289**	**77%**	**27**	**4**	**3**
Florida, 1	**365**	**70%**	**31**	**6**	**7**

Product and Portion Size	Calories	% Cal from Fat	Total Fat (g)	Bad Fat (g)	Net Carbs (g)
BABY FOODS, Cereals					
Beech-Nut Naturals					
Barley, 15g	60	0%	<1	0	11
Mixed, 15g	60	0%	1	0	10
Oatmeal, 15g	60	0%	1.5	0	10
Peaches Oatmeal & Bananas, 4 oz	100	0%	1.5	0	16
Rice, 15g	60	0%	0	0	12
BABY FOODS, Dinners, juniors					
Beech-Nut Stage 3					
Beef noodle, 1 jar	97	30%	3	1	11
Turkey & rice, 1 jar	95	15%	2	0	14
Gerber Third Foods					
Vegetables & chicken, 1 jar	90	19%	2	1	13
Vegetables & ham, 1 jar	102	28%	3	1	13
Vegetables & turkey, 1 jar	90	30%	3	1	11
Heinz Junior-3					
Chicken noodle, 1 jar	94	20%	2	1	13
Macaroni & cheese, 1 jar	104	29%	3	2	13

Product and Portion Size	Calories	% Cal from Fat	Total Fat (g)	Bad Fat (g)	Net Carbs (g)
Mixed vegetables, 1 jar	56	0%	0	0	13
Spaghetti, tomato & meat, 1 jar	116	12%	2	1	17
BABY FOODS, Dinners, strained					
Beech-Nut Stage 2					
Chicken noodle, 1 jar	75	28%	2	1	8
Sweet potato & chicken, 1 jar	84	26%	2	1	11
Earth's Best, vegetables & turkey, 1 jar	54	21%	1	0	7
Gerber Second Foods					
Beef noodle, 1 jar	71	32%	3	1	8
Broccoli & chicken, 1 jar	47	32%	2	0	1
Macaroni, tomato & beef, 1 jar	69	22%	2	1	11
Turkey & rice, 1 jar	59	22%	1	0	8
Heinz strained-2					
Apples & chicken, 1 jar	73	19%	2	0	10
Vegetables & bacon, 1 jar	80	38%	3	1	8
Vegetables & ham, 1 jar	57	33%	2	1	7

Product and Portion Size	Calories	% Cal from Fat	Total Fat (g)	Bad Fat (g)	Net Carbs (g)
BABY FOODS, Dinners, toddler					
Beech-Nut Table Time					
Beef stew, 1 jar	87	21%	2	1	7
Chicken, noodle, vegetables, 1 jar	112	23%	3	1	14
Spaghetti, tomato, meat, 1 jar	128	12%	2	0	18
Vegetable & turkey, 1 jar	136	38%	6	0	14
BABY FOODS, Fruit					
Beech-Nut Stage 1					
Applesauce, 2.5 oz	40	0%	0	0	8
Bananas, 2.5 oz	70	0%	0	0	15
Peaches, 2.5 oz	45	0%	0	0	8
Pears, 2.5 oz	50	0%	0	0	8
Beech-Nut Stage 2					
Applesauce, 4 oz	60	0%	0	0	13
Bartlett pears, 4 oz	70	0%	0	0	13
Cinnamon raisin pears w/apples, 4 oz	130	0%	0	0	31
Mango dessert, 4 oz	90	0%	0	0	19
Mixed fruit yogurt, 4 oz	100	0%	1	0	20

Product and Portion Size	Calories	% Cal from Fat	Total Fat (g)	Bad Fat (g)	Net Carbs (g)
Peaches & bananas, 4 oz	70	0%	0	0	15
Prunes w/pears, 4 oz	100	0%	0	0	24
Beech-Nut Stage 3					
Apples & cherries, 6 oz	90	0%	0	0	18
Applesauce, 6 oz	90	0%	0	0	18
Chiquita bananas & berries, 6 oz	170	0%	<1	0	37
Fruit dessert, 6 oz	100	0%	0	0	22
Beech-Nut Table Time					
Apple dices, 4 oz	50	0%	0	0	12
Peach dices, 4 oz	50	0%	0	0	11
BABY FOOD, Juices					
Beech-Nut					
Apple cherry (Naturals), 4 oz	60	0%	0	0	15
Apple (Naturals), 4 oz	60	0%	0	0	15
Guava nectar (Stage 2), 4 oz	60	0%	0	0	15
Mango nectar (Stage 2), 4 oz	70	0%	0	0	15
Mixed fruit (Naturals), 4 oz	80	0%	0	0	20

Product and Portion Size	Calories	% Cal from Fat	Total Fat (g)	Bad Fat (g)	Net Carbs (g)
BABY FOOD, Meat					
Beech-Nut Naturals					
Beef & broth, 2.5 oz	70	50%	4	0	0
Chicken & broth, 2.5 oz	50	45%	2.5	0	0
Lamb & broth, 2.5 oz	60	47%	3	0	0
Turkey & broth, 2.5 oz	90	50%	5	0	0
Veal & broth, 2.5 oz	50	36%	2	0	0
BABY FOOD, Snacks					
Beech-Nut, Arrowroot, 3 cookies	30	30%	1.5	0.5	5
Beech-Nut, Banana cookies, 1 cookie	30	33%	1.5	0.5	5
Beech-Nut, Biter biscuits, 1	40	22%	1	0	8
Beech-Nut, Cheese crackers, 7 crackers	30	33%	1	0.5	5
BABY FOOD, Vegetables (Beech-Nut)					
Butternut squash (Stage 1), 2.5 oz	30	0%	0	0	6
Butternut squash (Stage 2), 4 oz	45	0%	0	0	9
Carrots & peas (Stage 2), 4 oz	50	0%	0	0	7
Carrots & peas (Stage 3), 6 oz	70	0%	0	0	11
Corn & sweet potatoes (Stage 2), 4 oz	90	0%	0	0	17

Product and Portion Size	Calories	% Cal from Fat	Total Fat (g)	Bad Fat (g)	Net Carbs (g)
Country garden vegetables (Stage 2), 4 oz	50	0%	0	0	7
Green beans, corn & rice (Stage 3), 6 oz	90	10%	1	0	13
Pasta vegetable medley (1st Advantage), 4 oz	100	54%	6	0	9
Sweet potato soufflé, 4 oz	160	31%	7	0	19
Sweet potato & apples (Stage 2), 4 oz	70	0%	0	0	15
Tender golden sweet potatoes (Stage 2), 4 oz	70	0%	0	0	16
Tender sweet carrots (Stage 1), 2.5 oz	30	0%	0	0	5
Tender sweet peas (Stage 1), 2.5 oz	40	0%	0	0	5
Tender sweet peas (Stage 2), 4 oz	70	0%	0	0	9
Tender young green beans (Stage 2), 4 oz	45	0%	0	0	6
BACON					
Hormel, Canadian, 56g	68	38%	3	1	1
Oscar Mayer, center cut, ½ oz	50	70%	4	2	0
Oscar Mayer, hearty thick cut, ¾ oz	60	75%	5	1.5	0
Oscar Mayer, ready to serve, ½ oz	70	70%	5	2	0
Oscar Mayer, ready to serve, Canadian, 1¾ oz	60	25%	2	1	1
Oscar Mayer, traditional, ½ oz	70	71%	6	2	0

Product and Portion Size	Calories	% Cal from Fat	Total Fat (g)	Bad Fat (g)	Net Carbs (g)
BACON SUBSTITUTE					
Morningstar, 2 strips	60	72%	4.5	0.5	2
Yves, Canadian veggie bacon, 4g	80	6%	0.5	0	0
BAGELS					
Lenders, blueberry, 4"	264	6%	2	0	51
Pepperidge Farm, cinnamon-raisin, 1	270	3%	1	0	54
Pepperidge Farm, plain, 1	260	3%	1	0	51
Pepperidge Farm, whole wheat, 1	250	6%	1.5	0	43
Sara Lee					
Apple cinnamon, 1 4-oz	310	5%	1.5	0	61
Banana walnut, 1 4-oz	350	17%	7	2	57
Blueberry Jr., 1	70	0%	0	0	14
Blueberry toaster size, 1	160	3%	0.5	0	33
Cinnamon raisin, toaster size, 1	160	3%	0.5	0	32
Cranberry orange, 1 4-oz	310	5%	1.5	0	61
Heart healthy, 100% whole wheat, 1	220	7%	1.5	0	41
Honey wheat, toaster size, 1	250	4%	1	0	46
Onion, deluxe, 1	260	4%	1	0	49

Product and Portion Size	Calories	% Cal from Fat	Total Fat (g)	Bad Fat (g)	Net Carbs (g)
Onion, toaster size, 1	160	3%	1	0	32
Plain, toaster size, 1	160	3%	0.5	0	32
Sundried tomato & basil, 1	300	3%	1.5	0	59
BANANA, raw, 1 7"	105	0%	0	0	24
Banana chips, 1 oz	147	55%	9	8	14
BARBEQUE SAUCE					
Heinz Jack Daniels Tennessee, 2 Tbs	45	0%	0	0	9
Heinz Jack Daniels, steak sauce, 1 oz	19	0%	0	0	4
Hunts, original, bold, 2 Tbs	60	0%	0	0	14
Hunts, honey hickory, 2 Tbs	60	0%	0	0	14
Kraft, hickory smoke, 2 Tbs	40	0%	0	0	9
Kraft, original, 2 Tbs	40	0%	0	0	11
Kraft, thick spicy brown sugar, 2 Tbs	60	0%	0	0	15
BARLEY, cooked, 1 cup	193	0%	0	0	38
BASS, cooked, dry heat, 3 oz	105	24%	3	1	0
BEANS, baked					
B&M, maple flavor, ½ cup	145	6%	1	0	22
Bush's, Boston recipe, ½ cup	150	6%	1	0	26

Product and Portion Size	Calories	% Cal from Fat	Total Fat (g)	Bad Fat (g)	Net Carbs (g)
Campbell's, pork 'n beans, ½ cup	140	8%	1.5	0.5	18
Campbell's, brown sugar & bacon, ½ cup	160	14%	2.5	0.5	22
S&W, country BBQ, ½ cup	140	0%	0.5	0	22
S&W, honey mustard, ½ cup	140	3%	0.5	0	22
S&W, sweet bacon, ½ cup	140	0%	0.5	0	23
Van Camp's, bacon & brown sugar, ½ cup	140	6%	1	0	24
BEANS, other					
Adzuki, fresh, cooked w/salt, 1 cup	294	0%	0	0	40
Black, fresh, cooked w/salt, 1 cup	227	0%	0	0	26
Great northern, cooked w/salt, 1 cup	209	0%	1	0	24
Navy, cooked w/salt, 1 cup	255	0%	1	0	28
Eden organic, Adzuki, ½ cup	110	0%	0	0	14
Eden organic, black, ½ cup	110	9%	1	0	12
Eden organic, kidney, ½ cup	100	0%	0	0	8
Eden organic, navy, ½ cup	110	0%	0	0	13
Eden organic, pinto, ½ cup	110	9%	1	0	12
Eden organic, soybean (black), ½ cup	120	42%	6	1	1
S&W, black, ½ cup	70	0%	0	0	11

Product and Portion Size	Calories	% Cal from Fat	Total Fat (g)	Bad Fat (g)	Net Carbs (g)
S&W, kidney, ½ cup	100	5%	0.5	0	17
S&W, white, ½ cup	80	6%	0.5	0	13
BEEF					
Bottom sirloin, lean & fat, roasted, 3 oz	177	46%	9	3	0
Bottom sirloin, lean, selected, roasted, 3 oz	153	35%	6	3	0
Brisket, lean & fat, choice, braised, flat half, 3 oz	186	44%	9	3	0
Brisket, lean, choice, braised, flat half, 3 oz	180	30%	6	3	0
Chuck arm pot roast, lean & fat, braised, choice, 3 oz	264	58%	18	6	0
Chuck arm pot roast, lean, braised, choice, 3 oz	180	33%	7	2	0
Chuck blade roast, lean & fat, choice, braised, 3 oz	296	67%	22	9	0
Chuck blade roast, lean, choice, braised, 3 oz	225	51%	12	5	0
Chuck shoulder, lean & fat, choice, grilled, 3 oz	156	40%	7	3	0
Chuck shoulder, lean, choice, grilled, 3 oz	155	38%	7	2	0
Corned beef brisket, cooked, 3 oz	213	69%	16	5	0
Filet mignon, lean & fat, broiled, 3 oz	270	67%	20	8	0
Filet mignon, lean, broiled, 3 oz	197	48%	11	4	0
Ground, 70% lean, patty, pan broiled, 3 oz	202	59%	13	5	0
Ground, 80% lean, patty, baked, 3 oz	204	54%	12	5	0

Product and Portion Size	Calories	% Cal from Fat	Total Fat (g)	Bad Fat (g)	Net Carbs (g)
Ground, 95% lean, patty, baked, 3 oz	148	33%	5	2	0
Liver, pan fried, 3 oz	142	24%	4	1	0
London broil, lean & fat, choice, grilled, 3 oz	162	40%	7	3	0
Prime rib, lean & fat, choice, roasted, 3 oz	305	73%	25	10	0
Rib eye, lean & fat, select, broiled, 3 oz	196	49%	12	3	0
Rib eye, lean, select, broiled, 3 oz	153	29%	6	3	0
Round, bottom, lean & fat, choice, roasted, 3 oz	168	43%	9	3	0
Round, bottom, lean, choice, roasted, 3 oz	157	38%	6	2	0
Short loin, porterhouse, lean & fat, choice, broiled, 3 oz	241	64%	17	6	0
Short loin, porterhouse, lean, choice, broiled, 3 oz	190	52%	11	4	0
Top sirloin, lean & fat, choice, broiled, 3 oz	186	44%	9	3	0
Top sirloin, lean, choice, broiled, 3 oz	160	31%	6	2	0
BEEF SUBSTITUTES					
Amy's Kitchen, All American burger, 1	120	21%	3	0	12
Amy's Kitchen, California veg burger, 1	140	32%	5	0.5	15
Amy's Kitchen, Chicago veg burger, 1	160	28%	5	1.5	17
Amy's Kitchen, Texas veg burger, 1	120	21%	2.5	0	11
Boca Burgers					

Product and Portion Size	Calories	% Cal from Fat	Total Fat (g)	Bad Fat (g)	Net Carbs (g)
Grilled, All-American, 1	90	28%	3	1	1
Grilled, vegetable burger, 1	70	14%	1	0	2
Organic cheeseburger, 1	120	33%	4.5	2	4
Organic garden vegetable, 1	130	19%	3	0	5
Organic original, 1	100	5%	1	0	3
Organic roasted garlic, 1	130	19%	3	0.5	5
Organic vegan, 1	100	20%	2.5	0	5
Roasted garlic, 1	70	21%	1.5	0	2
Roasted onion, 1	70	14%	1	0	3
Morningstar Farms					
Grillers, vegan, 1	100	25%	2.5	0.5	3
Grillers, prime veggie, 1	170	47%	9	1	2
Garden veggie, 1	100	25%	2.5	0.5	5
Mushroom lover's burger, 1	110	45%	6	1	7
Spicy black bean, 1	140	25%	4	0.5	12
Steak strips, 12 strips	140	18%	3	0.5	22
Worthington (canned)					
Redi-Burger patties, ⅝"	120	21%	2.5	0.5	3

Product and Portion Size	Calories	% Cal from Fat	Total Fat (g)	Bad Fat (g)	Net Carbs (g)
Tender Rounds, 6 pcs	120	33%	4.5	0.5	5
Vege-Burger, ¼ cup	60	12%	0.5	0	0
Vegetarian burger, ¼ cup	70	21%	1.5	0	2
Worthington (frozen)					
Dinner roast, ¾" slice	180	56%	11	1.5	3
Meatless corned beef, 3 slices	140	57%	9	1	5
Meatless smoked beef, 3 slices	130	46%	7	1	6
Swiss Stake, 1 pc	130	38%	6	1	6
Yves					
Good veggie burger, 1	111	32%	4	0	9
Prime veggie burger, 1	120	30%	4	0	8
Veggie bistro burger, 1	140	32%	5	0	10
Veggie ground round, Mexican, 55g	85	26%	2.5	0	8
Veggie ground round, original, 55g	58	6%	0	0	10
Veggie "neatballs," 60g	74	24%	2	0	11
BEER, regular, 12 oz	153	0%	0	0	13
Lite, 12 oz	103	0%	0	0	6

Product and Portion Size	Calories	% Cal from Fat	Total Fat (g)	Bad Fat (g)	Net Carbs (g)
BEETS, fresh, boiled, sliced, ½ cup	37	0%	0	0	6
Del Monte, canned, sliced, ½ cup	35	0%	0	0	6
Del Monte, pickled, ½ cup	80	0%	0	0	17
BISCUITS, box/mix (Bisquick)					
Complete buttermilk, ⅓ cup mix	150	40%	7	5	20
Complete cheese garlic, ⅓ cup mix	160	44%	7	5	21
Heart smart, ⅓ cup mix	140	18%	2.5	0	26
Honey butter, ⅓ cup mix	160	38%	6	4.5	22
Original, ⅓ cup mix	160	31%	6	3	22
BISCUITS, refrigerated (Pillsbury)					
Country, 3 biscuits	150	10%	2	0	28
Freezer to Oven, buttermilk, 1	180	44%	9	6.5	20
Freezer to Oven, cheddar garlic, 1	190	47%	10	7.5	19
Freezer to Oven, southern, 1	180	44%	9	6.5	20
Grands, butter tastin', 1	190	42%	9	6	25
Grands, crescent, 1	270	48%	15	8	27
Grands, extra rich, 1	210	43%	10	7.5	25
Grands, flaky layers, buttermilk, 1	190	42%	9	5.5	23

Product and Portion Size	Calories	% Cal from Fat	Total Fat (g)	Bad Fat (g)	Net Carbs (g)
Golden layers, flaky, 1	110	36%	4.5	2.5	14
Microwave butter tastin', 1	200	45%	10	6.5	23
BLACKBERRIES, fresh, 1 cup	62	10%	1	0	6
BLUEBERRIES, fresh, 1 cup	83	0%	0	0	18
Cascadian Farm, frozen, 1 cup	70	14%	1	0	13
Dole, frozen, 1 cup	70	7%	1	0	13
Dole, frozen, wild, 1 cup	70	0%	0	0	17
BLUEFISH, baked, 3 oz	**135**	**31%**	**5**	**1**	**0**
BOK CHOY, cooked, shredded, 1 cup	20	0%	0	0	1
BOLOGNA					
Louis Rich, turkey bologna, 1 slice	52	63%	4	1	1
Oscar Mayer, beef, 1 slice	88	83%	8	4	1
Oscar Mayer, beef light, 1 slice	56	66%	4	2	2
Oscar Mayer, fat free, 1 slice	20	10%	0	0	2
BOULLION/BROTH					
College Inn					
Beef, 1 cup	25	40%	1	0	0
Beef, French onion style, 1 cup	15	0%	0	0	0

Product and Portion Size	Calories	% Cal from Fat	Total Fat (g)	Bad Fat (g)	Net Carbs (g)
Chicken, 99% f-f, 1 cup	15	66%	1	0	0
Chicken w/lemon & herb, 1 cup	15	66%	1	0	0
Garden vegetable, 1 cup	25	0%	0	0	6
Turkey, 1 cup	20	50%	1	0	0
HerbOx, chicken, regular, 1 cube	5	0%	0	0	0
HerbOx, chicken, sodium-free, 1 cube	10	0%	0	0	2
Imagine					
Organic beef broth, 8 oz	20	50%	1	0	1
Organic free range chicken, 8 oz	10	0%	0	0	1
Organic low-sodium vegetable broth, 8 oz	20	0%	0	0	2
Organic no chicken broth, 8 oz	10	0%	0	0	2
Organic vegetable broth, 8 oz	20	0%	0	0	2
Tyson beef, 1 cube	4	0%	0	0	0
Tyson chicken, 1 cube	4	0%	0	0	0
BRAZIL NUTS, unblanched, dried, 1 oz	**185**	**92%**	**4**	**0**	**1**
BREAD					
Arnold					
Carb country 100% whole wheat, 1 slice	60	10%	1.5	0	5

Product and Portion Size	Calories	% Cal from Fat	Total Fat (g)	Bad Fat (g)	Net Carbs (g)
Stone ground 100% whole wheat, 1 slice	70	15%	1.5	0	10
Stone ground, multigrain, 1 slice	70	10%	1	0	11
Whole grain classics, 12-grain, 1 slice	110	20%	2	0	17
Whole grain classics, 100% whole wheat, 1 slice	90	10%	1	0	15
Country classics, oatnut, 1 slice	110	20%	2	0	18
Country classics, oat bran, 1 slice	100	10%	1	0	17
Raisin cinnamon, 1 slice	100	20%	2	0	16
Real Jewish rye, 1 slice	90	15%	1.5	0	14
Earth Grains					
Buttermilk, 1 slice	110	14%	1.5	0	19
Honey wheat berry, 1 slice	100	5%	0.5	0	19
Honey whole grain, 1 slice	120	14%	1.5	0	19
Oat & nut, 1 slice	120	17%	2.5	0.5	19
Potato, 1 slice	110	9%	1	0	19
100% multigrain, 1 slice	110	9%	1.5	0	14
100% whole wheat extra fiber, 1 slice	110	9%	1.5	0	15
Oroweat					
7-grain, 1 slice	100	10%	1	0	19

Product and Portion Size	Calories	% Cal from Fat	Total Fat (g)	Bad Fat (g)	Net Carbs (g)
12-grain, 1 slice	110	13%	1.5	0	19
Buttermilk, country, 1 slice	100	10%	1	0	18
Healthnut, 1 slice	100	20%	2	0	16
Honey fiber whole grain, 1 slice	80	13%	1	0	12
Jewish rye, 1 slice	80	8%	1	0	13
Oatnut, 1 slice	100	15%	1.5	0	17
Potato, country, 1 slice	100	10%	1	0	19
Russian rye, 1 slice	80	8%	1	0	12
White, country, 1 slice	110	13%	1.5	0	19
Whole grain nut, 1 slice	90	17%	1.5	0	15
Whole wheat, 1 slice	100	10%	1	0	16
Pepperidge Farm					
7-grain light, 3 slices	130	45%	1	0	22
Carb style 100% whole wheat, 1 slice	60	10%	1.5	0	5
Cracked wheat thin, 1 slice	70	13%	1	0	12
Deli swirl, 1 slice	80	10%	1	0	13
Hearty white, 1 slice	120	15%	1.5	0.5	21
Honey whole wheat, 1 slice	110	15%	2	0.5	17

Product and Portion Size	Calories	% Cal from Fat	Total Fat (g)	Bad Fat (g)	Net Carbs (g)
Multigrain, whole grain, 1 slice	120	20%	2	0	17
Pumpernickel, 1 slice	80	10%	1	0	14
Sara Lee					
Classic wheat, 1 slice	70	12%	1	0	11
Country potato, 1 slice	100	8%	1	0	20
Cracked wheat, 1 slice	110	8%	1	0	20
Delightful white, 2 slices	90	9%	1	0	14
Heart healthy multigrain, 1 slice	100	9%	1	0	17
Honey nut & oat, 1 slice	113	12%	1.5	0	19
Honey wheat, 1 slice	110	8%	1	0	21
Honey white, 1 slice	100	4%	0.5	0.5	22
Sheepherder country, 1 slice	110	8%	1	0	20
Sourdough, 1 slice	110	8%	1	0	22
Stroehmann					
Dutch country, 12-grain, 1 slice	100	15%	1.5	0	18
Dutch country, honey cracked wheat, 1 slice	90	10%	1	0	17
Dutch country, potato, 1 slice	100	15%	1.5	0	18
Family grains, 100% whole wheat, 1 slice	80	19%	1.5	0	11

Product and Portion Size	Calories	% Cal from Fat	Total Fat (g)	Bad Fat (g)	Net Carbs (g)
Family grains, king white, 2 slices	130	12%	1.5	0	24
Family grains, multigrain, 1 slice	80	15%	1.5	0	12
Family grains, oat & honey, 1 slice	80	15%	1.5	0	12
Wonder					
Beefsteak, soft rye, 1 slice	70	10%	1	0	13
Kids sandwich, 1 slice	60	5%	0.5	0	10
Light wheat, 2 slices	80	10%	0.5	0	13
Stone ground 100% whole wheat, 1 slice	80	10%	1	0	12
Whole grain white, 2 slices	130	20%	2	0.5	21
BREAD—Frozen (Pepperidge Farm)					
Garlic, 2.5" slice	160	31%	6	1.5	21
Texas toast, garlic, 1 slice	150	31%	7	5	16
Texas toast, mozzarella & Monterey jack, 1 slice	160	38%	6	1.5	19
BREADCRUMBS					
Devonsheer, plain, ⅛ cup	110	13%	1.5	0	18
Progresso, plain, ¼ cup	110	14%	1.5	0.5	19
Progresso, garlic & herb, ¼ cup	110	14%	1.5	0.5	19
Progresso, Italian style, ¼ cup	110	14%	1.5	0.5	19

Product and Portion Size	Calories	% Cal from Fat	Total Fat (g)	Bad Fat (g)	Net Carbs (g)
BROCCOLI, fresh, boiled, ½ cup chopped	27	11%	0	0	3
Frozen, Birds Eye					
Chopped, ¾ cup	30	0%	0	0	2
Florets, 1 cup	30	0%	0	0	2
Tender cuts, 1 cup	30	0%	0	0	2
w/cheese sauce, ½ cup	90	50%	5	3	7
w/beans, peppers, onion, 1 cup	30	0%	0	0	3
w/corn & peppers, ¾ cup	60	15%	1	0	10
w/peppers, onion, mushrooms, 1 cup	30	0%	0	0	3
w/cauliflower & peppers, 1 cup	25	0%	0	0	2
Frozen, Green Giant					
Spears in butter, 4 oz	50	40%	2	1	4
w/cauliflower, carrots, cheese, ⅔ cup	60	42%	2.5	1	6
w/cheese, ⅔ cup	60	38%	2.5	1	5
w/three cheese sauce, ⅔ cup	50	42%	2.5	1	6
w/zesty cheese, ¾ cup	60	25%	2	0.5	7
BRUSSELS SPROUTS, fresh, boiled, ½ cup	28	11%	0	0	4
Birds Eye, frozen, 10 sprouts	45	0%	0	0	5

Product and Portion Size	Calories	% Cal from Fat	Total Fat (g)	Bad Fat (g)	Net Carbs (g)
Birds Eye, w/cauliflower & carrots, 1 cup	40	0%	0	0	5
Green Giant, w/butter sauce, ½ cup	70	14%	1	0.5	7
BULGUR, cooked, 1 cup	151	0%	0	0	26
BUTTER, regular, salted, 1 Tbs	100	100%	11	7	0
Whipped, salted, 1 Tbs	66	100%	8	5	0
BUTTERMILK, lowfat, 1 cup	98	19%	2	1	12
CABBAGE					
Green, raw, shredded, ½ cup	8	0%	0	0	1
Green, boiled, no salt, ½ cup shredded	16	18%	0	0	2
Napa, cooked, 1 cup	13	15%	0	0	2
Red, raw, chopped, 1 cup	28	0%	0	0	5
Red, boiled, shredded, 1 cup	44	5%	0	0	6
Savoy, raw, shredded, 1 cup	19	5%	0	0	2
Savoy, boiled, shredded, 1 cup	35	3%	0	0	4
CAKE, bakery-type					
Entenmann's, All-butter loaf, ⅙ cake	220	36%	9	6	31
Entenmann's, Caramel mocha, ⅙ cake	260	42%	12	5	35
Entenmann's, Cinnamon crumb, ⅑ cake	320	41%	14	5	44

Product and Portion Size	Calories	% Cal from Fat	Total Fat (g)	Bad Fat (g)	Net Carbs (g)
Entenmann's Coffee house crunch, 1/6 cake	290	45%	14	5	38
Entenmann's, Filled chocolate chip crumb, 1/9 cake	390	49%	21	8	48
Entenmann's, French crumb, 1/8 cake	210	43%	10	5	28
Entenmann's, Louisiana crumb, 1/9 cake	330	39%	14	4	48
Entenmann's pina colada, 1/6 cake	290	48%	15	7	36
CAKE, boxed mixes (mix only) Betty Crocker					
Angel food confetti, 1/12 cake	150	0%	0	0	34
Angel food white, 1/12 cake	140	0%	0	0	32
Brownie, fudge, chewy, 1/20	110	14%	1.5	1	24
Brownie, fudge, low fat, 1/18 prep.	130	15%	2.5	1.5	27
Brownie, supreme, frosted, 1/18	150	17%	3	2	29
Brownie, supreme, peanut butter, 1/20 pkg	130	19%	3	2.5	23
Brownie, supreme, turtle, 1/20 pkg	120	21%	2.5	0.5	23
Complete Desserts, hot fudge cake, 1/6 pkg	430	26%	13	6	75
Gingerbread cake & cookie mix, 1/8 pkg	210	24%	5	3	39
Pineapple upside down cake, 1/6 cake	350	23%	9	5.5	65

Product and Portion Size	Calories	% Cal from Fat	Total Fat (g)	Bad Fat (g)	Net Carbs (g)
Pound cake, 1/8 cake	240	25%	7	4	45
Quick bread, banana, 1/12 cake	130	19%	2.5	1.5	25
Quick bread, cinnamon streusel, 1/14 cake	160	22%	4	2	28
Quick bread, cranberry orange, 1/12 cake	150	17%	3	1	29
Quick bread, lemon poppy seed, 1/12 cake	130	15%	2.5	1	25
Super Moist					
Butter pecan, 1/12 cake	170	18%	3	2.5	35
Butter recipe chocolate, 1/12 cake	170	15%	3	2	33
Carrot, 1/12 cake	200	13%	3	2	42
Chocolate fudge, 1/12 cake	170	15%	3	1.5	34
Cinnamon swirl, 1/12 cake	200	15%	3.5	2	42
French vanilla, 1/12 cake	170	18%	3	2.5	35
German chocolate, 1/12 cake	170	18%	3	2.5	34
Lemon, 1/12 cake	170	18%	3	2.5	41
Party rainbow chip, 1/10 cake	210	19%	4.5	2.5	41
Pineapple, 1/10 cake	170	18%	3	2.5	35
Spice, 1/12 cake	170	18%	3.5	2.5	35

Product and Portion Size	Calories	% Cal from Fat	Total Fat (g)	Bad Fat (g)	Net Carbs (g)
Strawberry, 1/12 cake	170	18%	3	2.5	35
Triple chocolate fudge, 1/12 cake	180	20%	4	2.5	34
Yellow, 1/12 cake	170	18%	3	2.5	35
CAKE, Frozen					
Mrs. Smith's all butter pound, ¼ cake	300	47%	16	9	34
Mrs. Smith's carrot cake, ⅙ cake	300	47%	16	4.5	35
Pepperidge Farm, coconut, ⅛ cake	250	40%	11	6	37
Pepperidge Farm, chocolate fudge, ⅛ cake	250	40%	11	6.5	30
Pepperidge Farm, chocolate fudge stripe, ⅛ cake	250	42%	13	6.5	30
Pepperidge Farm, vanilla, ⅛ cake	250	40%	11	6	34
CAKE, Snack					
Drake's, coffee cake, 2	280	39%	12	5	39
Drake's, Devil Dogs, 1	170	35%	7	4	25
Drake's, Devil Dogs, reduced fat, 1	160	21%	4	2	28
Drake's, Funny Bones, peanut butter, 2	310	45%	16	9.5	36
Drake's, Yodels, 2	280	46%	14	10	35
Hostess, chocolate cupcakes, 1	180	40%	6	2.5	29
Hostess, Ho Ho's, caramel, 3 cakes	380	40%	17	13.5	51

Product and Portion Size	Calories	% Cal from Fat	Total Fat (g)	Bad Fat (g)	Net Carbs (g)
Hostess, Twinkies, 1	150	27%	4.5	2.5	27
Tastykake					
Chocolate cupcakes, single serve, 3 cakes	310	29%	10	5	52
Chocolate cupcakes, cream filled, single serve, 3 cakes	370	34%	14	6.5	57
Chocolate Junior, single serve, 1	340	32%	12	6	54
Coconut Junior, single serve, 1	340	32%	12	2.5	54
Fudge nut brownies, ½ brownie	150	35%	7	1.5	27
Glazed honey bun, family pack, 1 bun	330	51%	18	11	37
Kandy Kake, Boston Kreme, 2 cakes	150	45%	9	4.5	24
Kandy Kake, mint, 2 cakes	170	44%	9	5	24
Kreamies, banana, 1 cake	170	41%	8	4	25
Krimpets, butterscotch, 2 cakes	210	29%	6	3	37
Krimpets, jelly, 2 cakes	180	20%	4	1	34
Raspberry koffee kake, low-fat, 2 cakes	170	13%	2.5	0.5	35
Snowballs, 1	210	29%	7	2.5	36
CANDY					
Almond Joy (Hershey), 45g	220	50%	12	8	25
Bit-O-Honey (Nestle), 6 pcs	160	17%	3	2	32

Product and Portion Size	Calories	% Cal from Fat	Total Fat (g)	Bad Fat (g)	Net Carbs (g)
Caramello, 6 blocks	200	40%	9	6	26
Chocolate bar, dairy milk (Cadbury), 10 blocks	220	50%	12	8	23
Chocolate bar, Fruit n Nut (Cadbury), 10 blocks	200	45%	10	5	24
Chocolate bar (Hershey), 43g	230	52%	13	9	24
Chocolate bar, pure dark (Hershey), 3 blocks	210	57%	13	8	16
Chocolate bar, milk w/almonds, 41g	230	52%	14	6	20
Chocolate bar, w/caramel (Hershey N' More), 25g	110	38%	5	4	15
Chocolate bar, Cookies n' crème (Hershey), 43g	230	48%	12	6	26
5th Avenue	280	46%	14	5	33
Goobers, 10 pcs	51	55%	3	1	4
Heath Toffee bar, 39g	220	55%	13	7	24
Kisses (Hershey), 9 pcs	230	52%	13	8	23
Kisses, Hugs, 9 pcs	210	52%	12	7	23
Kisses w/peanut butter, 9 pcs	230	56%	14	7	20
Kit Kat, 1 4-pc bar	220	45%	11	7	26
Kit Kat, white, 1 4-pc bar	220	50%	12	8	26
Krackel, 41g	210	43%	10	6	27
Milk Duds, 13 pcs	180	33%	7	3.5	28

Product and Portion Size	Calories	% Cal from Fat	Total Fat (g)	Bad Fat (g)	Net Carbs (g)
M&Ms, 1.69 oz	240	38%	10	6	33
M&M, peanut, 1.74 oz	250	48%	13	5	28
M&M, almond, 1.31 oz	200	50%	11	3.5	19
Milky Way, 2.05 oz	260	35%	10	7	40
Milky Way Midnight, 1.76 oz	220	32%	8	5	35
Mounds, 49g	240	50%	13	10	27
Mr. Goodbar, 49g	270	52%	16	7	25
Pay Day, 52g	250	48%	13	2.5	26
Raisinets, 1 oz	116	34%	4	2	20
Reese's NutRageous, 51g	280	50%	16	5	25
Reese's peanut butter & white chocolate, 42g	230	52%	13	4.5	21
Reese's Pieces, 43g	220	45%	11	7	25
Rolo, 48g	210	38%	9	7	31
S'mores, 46g	230	43%	11	6	30
Skor, 39g	210	52%	12	7	23
Symphony, milk chocolate, 42g	230	52%	13	8	23
Take 5, 42g	210	43%	10	5	25
Tootsie Roll, 6 pcs	155	8%	1	0	35

Product and Portion Size	Calories	% Cal from Fat	Total Fat (g)	Bad Fat (g)	Net Carbs (g)
Twix, 1 oz	155	55%	9	1	15
Twizzlers, strawberry, 2.5 oz	249	6%	2	0	57
Whatchamacallit	220	45%	11	8	27
Whoppers, 21g	100	30%	3.5	3	16
York peppermint patty, 39g	160	16%	3	1.5	31
CANTALOUPE, raw, ½ medium melon	94	4%	<1	0	19
CARROTS					
Raw, 1 large 7–8.5"	30	0%	0	0	5
Cooked, no salt, ½ cup slices	27	0%	0	0	4
Birds Eye, frozen, whole baby, ⅔ cup	35	9%	9	9	5
Birds Eye, frozen, sliced, ⅔ cup	35	0%	0	0	5
Del Monte canned, ½ cup	35	0%	0	0	5
Del Monte canned, honey glazed, ½ cup	70	0%	0	0	17
CARROT JUICE, Odwalla, 8 oz	70	0%	0	0	14
Hain w/lutein, 8 oz	80	6%	0.5	0	16
CASABA MELON, raw, 1 cup cubes	48	2%	0	0	9
CASHEWS, dry roast, no salt, 1 oz	**162**	**68%**	**13**	**3**	**8**
CASHEW BUTTER, Maranatha, 2 Tbs	**190**	**74%**	**15**	**3**	**9**

Product and Portion Size	Calories	% Cal from Fat	Total Fat (g)	Bad Fat (g)	Net Carbs (g)
CAULIFLOWER, raw, 1 cup	25	4%	0	0	2
Boiled, no salt, 1 cup	28	14%	0	0	1
Birds Eye, frozen, florets, 4 pcs	25	0%	0	0	3
Birds Eye, cauliflower & garlic sauce, 1¼ cup	60	0%	4	1	4
Birds Eye, cauliflower, carrots & snow pea pods, 1 cup	30	0%	0	0	4
Green Giant, cauliflower & cheese sauce, ½ cup	50	40%	2.5	1	5
Green Giant, cauliflower & 3 cheese sauce, ½ cup prep.	45	44%	2	0.5	5
CAVIAR, red & black, 1 oz	71	65%	5	1	1
CELERY, raw, 7–8" stalk	6	17%	0	0	0
Chopped, 1 cup	14	7%	0	0	1
CEREAL, cold/dry, ready-to-eat					
Arrowhead Mills					
Amaranth flakes, 1 cup	140	7%	2	0	23
Bran flakes, 1 cup	110	9%	1	0	17
Kamut flakes, 1 cup	120	8%	1	0.5	23
Multigrain flakes, 1 cup	170	9%	2	0	30
Organic nature Os, 1 cup	130	15%	2	0.5	23
Puffed corn, 1 cup	60	8%	1	0	10

Product and Portion Size	Calories	% Cal from Fat	Total Fat (g)	Bad Fat (g)	Net Carbs (g)
Puffed millet, 1 cup	60	8%	0.5	0	10
Rice flakes, sweetened, 1 cup	180	6%	1	0	39
Sweetened shredded wheat, 1 cup	200	5%	1	0	37
Barbara's Bakery					
Alpen, original, ⅔ cup	200	13%	3	0	37
Brown Rice Crisps, 1 cup	120	4%	1	0	24
Honey Nut O's, organic, ¾ cup	120	13%	2	0	22
Organic Wild Puffs, caramel, ¾ cup	110	9%	1	0	24
Puffins, original, ¾ cup	90	11%	1	0	18
Puffins, peanut butter, ¾ cup	110	18%	2	0.5	21
Shredded oats, 1¼ cup	220	11%	2.5	0.5	41
Soy Essence, ¾ cup	110	3%	0.5	0	20
General Mills					
Apple cinnamon Cheerios, ¾ cup	120	13%	1.5	0	24
Cheerios, 1 cup	110	14%	2	0	19
Cheerios, honey nut, ¾ cup	110	14%	1.5	0	20
Cheerios, multigrain, 1 cup	110	9%	1	0	20
Basic 4, 1 cup	202	12%	3	1	39

Product and Portion Size	Calories	% Cal from Fat	Total Fat (g)	Bad Fat (g)	Net Carbs (g)
Cinnamon Toast Crunch, ¾ cup	127	24%	3	1	23
Cocoa Puffs, 1 cup	117	8%	1	0	25
Corn Chex, 1 cup	112	2%	0	0	25
Corn Flakes, 1 cup	111	4%	0	0	25
Fiber One, ½ cup	60	12%	1	0	10
Frosted Wheaties, ¾ cup	112	3%	0	0	26
Golden Grahams, ¾ cup	112	8%	1	0	24
Kix, 1¼ cup	110	4%	1	0	25
Lucky Charms, ¾ cup	110	9%	1	0	21
Nature Valley Low-Fat Fruit Granola, ⅔ cup	212	11%	3	0	41
Oatmeal Crisp w/almonds, 1 cup	218	19%	5	1	38
Oatmeal Raisin crisp, 1 cup	204	9%	2	0	41
Raisin Nut Bran, 1 cup	209	19%	4	1	36
Rice Chex, 1¼ cup	117	3%	0	0	27
Total, whole grain, ¾ cup	97	6%	1	0	19
Total, corn flakes, 1⅓ cup	112	4%	0	0	25
Trix, 1 cup	117	9%	1	0	26
Wheaties, ¾ cup	100	5%	0.5	0	20

Product and Portion Size	Calories	% Cal from Fat	Total Fat (g)	Bad Fat (g)	Net Carbs (g)
Health Valley					
Corn Crunch-ems, 1 cup	110	0%	0	0	25
Date Almond Granola, low fat, ⅔ cup	180	6%	1	0	37
Heart Wise, 1 cup	**200**	**13%**	**3**	**0**	**31**
Organic Amaranth Flakes, ¾ cup	100	0%	0	0	20
Organic Blue Corn Flakes, ¾ cup	100	0%	0	0	20
Organic Oat Bran Flakes w/raisins, ¾ cup	110	0%	0	0	22
Original Soy Flakes, 1¼ cup	190	8%	1.5	0	30
Raisin Cinnamon Granola, low fat, ⅔ cup	180	6%	1	0	37
Slender, 1 cup	180	8%	1.5	0	31
Kashi					
Go Lean, ¾ cup	114	6%	1	0	15
Good Friends, ¾ cup	95	11%	1	0	18
Heart to Heart, ¾ cup	115	12%	2	0	20
Medley, ¾ cup	113	6%	1	0	23
Organic Promise, Autumn Wheat, 1 cup	181	6%	1	0	37
Organic Promise, Cranberry, 1 cup	92	9%	1	0	18
Organic Promise, Strawberry Fields, 1 cup	111	0%	0	0	27

Product and Portion Size	Calories	% Cal from Fat	Total Fat (g)	Bad Fat (g)	Net Carbs (g)
Seven in the Morning, 1 cup	207	7%	2	0	40
Kellogg's					
All-Bran Buds, ⅓ cup	70	7%	1	0	11
Apple Jacks, 1 cup	130	4%	0.5	0	29
Cocoa Krispies, ¾ cup	120	8%	1	0.5	26
Complete Oat Bran Flakes, ¾ cup	110	9%	1	0	19
Corn Flakes, 1 cup	101	0%	0	0	23
Corn Pops, 1 cup	117	1%	0	0	28
Cracklin' Oat Bran, ¾ cup	220	30%	7	3	29
Froot Loops, 1 cup	120	8%	1	0.5	27
Frosted Flakes, ¾ cup	120	0%	0	0	27
Frosted Mini Wheats, 24 bite-size biscuits	200	5%	1	0	42
Just Right Fruit & Nut, ¾ cup	200	10%	2	0	40
Low-Fat Granola w/raisins, ⅔ cup	201	12%	3	1	41
Mueslix, ⅔ cup	200	13%	3	0	36
Product 19, 1 cup	100	0%	0	0	24
Puffed Wheat, 1 oz	94	4%	0	0	20
Raisin Bran, 1 cup	190	8%	1.5	0	36

Product and Portion Size	Calories	% Cal from Fat	Total Fat (g)	Bad Fat (g)	Net Carbs (g)
Rice Krispies, 1¼ cup	120	0%	0	0	29
Rice Krispies Treat Cereal, ¾ cup	120	13%	1.5	0	26
Smart Start Antioxidants, 1 cup	190	3%	0.5	0	40
Smart Start Healthy Heart Maple Brown Sugar, 1¼ cup	230	13%	3	0.5	41
Special K, 1 cup	110	0%	0	0	21
Malt-O-Meal					
Apple-Cinnamon Toasty Os, ¾ cup	120	13%	1.5	0	23
Coco Roos, ¾ cup	120	13%	1.5	0	25
Colossal Crunch, ¾ cup	120	13%	1.5	0	26
Crispy Rice, 1¼ cup	130	0%	0	0	29
Frosted Flakes, ¾ cup	120	0%	0	0	27
Frosted Mini Spooners, 1 cup	190	5%	1	0	39
Honey Nut Toasty Os, 1 cup	110	9%	1.5	0	22
Marshmallow Mateys, 1 cup	120	8%	1	0	24
Raisin Bran, 1 cup	220	5%	1	0	40
Tootie Fruities, 1 cup	130	8%	1	0	27
Post					
Alpha Bits, 1 oz	110	14%	2	0	19

Product and Portion Size	Calories	% Cal from Fat	Total Fat (g)	Bad Fat (g)	Net Carbs (g)
Banana Nut Crunch, 2 oz	240	21%	6	0.5	39
Blueberry Morning Selects, 2 oz	230	11%	3	0	45
Bran Flakes, 1 oz	100	5%	0.5	0	19
Cocoa Pebbles, 1 oz	110	9%	1.5	1	23
Cranberry Almond Crunch Selects, 2 oz	220	14%	3	0	45
Fruit & Bran, 2 oz	200	15%	3	0	36
Golden Crisp, 1 oz	110	0%	0	0	24
Grape Nuts, 2 oz	200	5%	1	0	41
Grape Nut Flakes, 1 oz	110	9%	1	0	21
Great Grains Crunchy Pecans Selects, 2 oz	220	27%	6	1	34
Honey Bunches of Oats, Honey Roasted, 1 oz	120	13%	1.5	0	23
Honey Bunches of Oats, Strawberry, 1 oz	120	13%	2	0	25
Honey Comb, 1 oz	120	8%	1	0	25
Maple Pecan Crunch Selects, 2 oz	220	23%	6	2	33
Oreo Os, 1 oz	110	14%	2	0.5	21
Quaker					
Life, cinnamon, ¾ cup	120	13%	1.5	0	23
Life, honey graham, ¾ cup	120	13%	1.5	0	23

Product and Portion Size	Calories	% Cal from Fat	Total Fat (g)	Bad Fat (g)	Net Carbs (g)
Life, original, ¾ cup	120	13%	1.5	0	23
Mothers Peanut Butter Bumpers, 1 cup	130	19%	2.5	0.5	25
Mothers Toasted Oat Bran, ¾ cup	120	13%	1.5	0	21
CEREALS, hot					
Arrowhead Mills					
4 Grains plus Flax, ¼ cup	140	7%	1.5	0	19
Bear Mush, ¼ cup	150	6%	1	0	30
Bits O Barley, ¼ cup	160	5%	1	0	28
Instant maple Apple Spice, 1 packet	140	14%	2	0	23
Instant oatmeal, original, 1 packet	110	18%	2	0	17
Oat Flakes, ⅓ cup	130	15%	2	0.5	19
Rice and Shine, ¼ cup	150	6%	1	0	30
Yellow corn grits, ¼ cup	130	0%	0	0	29
Cream of Wheat					
Apple & cinnamon instant, 1 packet	130	0%	0	0	28
Cinnamon swirl, 1 packet	130	0%	0	0	27
Maple brown sugar, 1 packet	120	0%	0	0	26
Quaker					

Product and Portion Size	Calories	% Cal from Fat	Total Fat (g)	Bad Fat (g)	Net Carbs (g)
Instant, apples & cinnamon, 1 packet	130	11%	1.5	0.5	24
Instant, maple & brown sugar, 1 packet	160	13%	2	0	30
Multigrain hot cereal, ½ cup	130	8%	1	0	24
Nutrition for Women, golden brown sugar, 1 packet	160	15%	2.5	0.5	29
Nutrition for Women, vanilla cinnamon, 1 packet	160	13%	2	0.5	29
Oatmeal, Express baked apple, 1 cup	200	13%	2.5	0.5	38
Oatmeal, Express cinnamon roll, 1 cup	210	14%	3.5	0.5	38
Quick Oats, ½ cup dry	150	17%	3	0.5	23
CEREAL BARS					
Barbara's Bakery					
Fruit & yogurt bars, apple cinnamon, 1	150	17%	3	0	27
Fruit & yogurt bars, blueberry apple, 1	150	17%	3	0	28
Fruit & yogurt bars, cherry apple, 1	150	17%	3	0	28
Granola, carob chip, 1	80	19%	2	0	14
Granola, cinnamon & raisin, 1	80	25%	2	0	13
Granola, oats & honey, 1	80	25%	2	0	13
Granola, peanut butter, 1	80	38%	3	0	12
Multigrain, apple cinnamon, 1	120	13%	1.5	0	23

Product and Portion Size	Calories	% Cal from Fat	Total Fat (g)	Bad Fat (g)	Net Carbs (g)
Multigrain, cherry, 1	120	13%	1.5	0	23
Puffins, Cereal & Milk Bars, blueberry	140	11%	1.5	1	21
Puffins, Cereal & Milk Bars, French toast, 1	130	12%	1.5	1	21
Puffins, Cereal & Milk Bars, peanut butter choc chip, 1	140	25%	3.5	1.5	20
Cascadian Farm					
Granola, chocolate chip, 1	140	21%	3	1	24
Granola, fruit & nut, 1	140	25%	4	0.5	23
Granola, harvest berries, 1	130	12%	2	0	26
Granola, multigrain, 1	130	12%	2	0	26
Health Valley					
Apple Cobbler, 1	130	15%	2	0	26
Apricot fruit bar, fat free, 1	140	0%	0	0	32
Café Creations, cinnamon danish bar, 1	130	19%	2.5	0	25
Café Creations, chocolate raspberry, 1	130	19%	3	0	25
Fig cobbler cereal bar, 1	130	15%	2	0	26
Moist & Chewy Dutch apple granola, 1	100	10%	1	0	20
Peanut butter & grape bar, 1	130	19%	2.5	0	25
Raspberry granola bar, fat free, 1	140	0%	0	0	32

Product and Portion Size	Calories	% Cal from Fat	Total Fat (g)	Bad Fat (g)	Net Carbs (g)
Strawberry cobbler cereal bar, 1	130	15%	2	0	26
Kellogg's					
All-Bran brown sugar cinnamon bar, 1	130	19%	3	0.5	22
Cocoa Krispies cereal & milk bar, 1	100	25%	2.5	2	17
Nutri-Grain, apple cinnamon, 1	140	18%	3	0.5	25
Nutri-Grain, cherry, 1	140	18%	3	0.5	25
Nutri-Grain, mixed berry, 1	140	18%	3	0.5	25
Nutri-Grain, muffin bar, banana, 1	170	21%	4	0.5	29
Nutri-Grain, muffin bar, cinnamon & raisin, 1	170	21%	4	0.5	31
Nutri-Grain, yogurt bar, strawberry, 1	140	18%	3	0.5	25
Nutri-Grain, granola bar, honey oat & raisin, 1	140	18%	3	0.5	25
Nature Valley					
Apple Crisp, 1	140	21%	3.5	2	25
Banana nut, 1	90	30%	3.5	0.5	13
Maple brown sugar, 1	90	30%	3	0	14
Oats & honey, 1	90	28%	3	0	14
Peanut butter, 1	90	30%	3.5	0	14
Pecan crunch, 1	90	30%	3.5	0.5	13
Roasted almond, 1	90	30%	3.5	0.5	13

Product and Portion Size	Calories	% Cal from Fat	Total Fat (g)	Bad Fat (g)	Net Carbs (g)
Quaker					
Breakfast bar, strawberry, 1	130	19%	2.5	0.5	26
Cranberry orange muffin, 1	130	19%	2.5	0.5	25
Iced raspberry, 1	130	19%	2.5	0.5	25
CHEESE					
American (Alpine Lace), 1 slice	90	66%	6	4.5	1
American, 2% milk, singles (Kraft), 1 slice	50	48%	2.5	1.5	2
American, singles (Kraft), 1 slice	60	72%	4.5	2.5	1
American, Deli Delux (Kraft), 1 slice	80	80%	7	4	0
American (Land-O-Lakes), 1 oz	110	63%	9	6	0
American (Maggiore), 1 slice	89	71%	7	6	<1
American, burger, deli style (Sargento), 1 slice	70	75%	6	3.5	<1
Camembert, 1 oz	85	71%	7	4	0
Cheddar, reduced fat (Alpine Lace), 1 slice	90	69%	7	4.5	0
Cheddar, 2% milk, sharp (Kraft), singles, 1 slice	50	57%	3	2	0
Cheddar, 2% milk, sharp (Kraft), shredded, ¼ cup	80	66%	6	3.5	0
Cheddar, mild (Organic Valley), 1 oz	110	74%	9	6	0
Cheddar, sharp (Organic Valley), 1 oz	110	74%	9	6	0

Product and Portion Size	Calories	% Cal from Fat	Total Fat (g)	Bad Fat (g)	Net Carbs (g)
Cheddar, double, chef style (Sargento), ¼ cup	110	72%	9	5	1
Cheddar, natural mild cubes (Sargento), 7 cubes	120	75%	10	6	<1
Cheddar, sharp deli style, sliced (Sargento), 1 slice	80	73%	6	4	0
Colby (Organic Valley), 1 oz	110	73%	9	6	0
Colby, longhorn, pre-sliced (Sara Lee), 1 slice	109	74%	9	5	0
Colby, deli style, sliced (Sargento), 1 slice	80	74%	7	4	0
Colby, natural Colby jack cubes (Sargento), 7 cubes	110	76%	9	6	0
Cottage Cheese					
Breakstone, small curd, fat free, 5 oz	80	0%	0	0	8
Breakstone, large curd, 2%, 4 oz	90	22%	2.5	1.5	6
Breakstone, small curd, 4%, 4 oz	120	38%	5	3	6
Breakstone, Cottage Doubles, apples & cinnamon, 5.5 oz	140	14%	2.5	1.5	18
Breakstone, Cottage Doubles, blueberry, 5.5 oz	140	14%	2.5	1.5	18
Breakstone, Cottage Doubles, peach, 5.5 oz	130	15%	2	1.5	16
Breakstone, Cottage Doubles, strawberry, 5.5 oz	130	15%	2	1.5	17
Knudsen, free nonfat, ½ cup	80	0%	0	0	7
Knudsen, small curd, ½ cup	120	38%	5	3	5
Knudsen, small curd low fat (2%), ½ cup	100	20%	2.5	1.5	6

Product and Portion Size	Calories	% Cal from Fat	Total Fat (g)	Bad Fat (g)	Net Carbs (g)
Knudsen, Cottage Doubles, apples & cinnamon, 1 cont.	140	14%	2	1.5	18
Knudsen, Cottage Doubles, blueberry, 1 container	140	14%	2.5	1.5	17
Knudsen, Cottage Doubles, peach, 1 container	140	14%	2.5	1.5	17
Knudsen, Cottage Doubles, pineapple, 1 container	130	15%	2.5	1.5	17
Knudsen, Cottage Doubles, raspberry, 1 container	150	13%	2.5	1.5	20
Knudsen, Cottage Doubles, strawberry, 1 container	140	14%	2.5	1.5	19
Organic Valley, organic, small curd, ½ cup	100	20%	2	1.5	4
Cream cheese (Philadelphia)					
Blueberry, 1.2 oz	90	78%	7	4.5	5
Fat free, 1 oz	30	0%	0	0	2
Garden vegetable, 1.2 oz	90	78%	8	5	2
Jalapeno light, 1.2 oz	60	67%	4.5	2.5	2
Original, 1 oz	100	90%	10	6	1
Neufchatel ⅓ less fat, 1 oz	70	86%	6	4	1
Peaches 'n cream, 1.2 oz	90	78%	7	4	5
Salmon, 1.2 oz	80	88%	8	4.5	2
Whipped, ¾ oz	60	83%	6	3.5	1
Whipped, chives, ¾ oz	60	83%	6	3.5	1

Product and Portion Size	Calories	% Cal from Fat	Total Fat (g)	Bad Fat (g)	Net Carbs (g)
Whipped, mixed berry, ¾ oz	70	71%	5	3	3
Edam, specialty (Sara Lee), 1 oz	105	69%	8	5	0
Edam (Boar's Head), 1 oz	91	69%	7	4.5	0
Feta, mild (Athenos), ¼ cup	91	69%	7	4.5	1
Feta (Boar's Head), 1 oz	60	60%	4	2.5	1
Feta crumbles (Organic Valley), 1 oz	60	62%	4	2.5	<1
Goat (Alta Dena), 1 oz	104	69%	8	5	1
Goat (Chavrie), 1.1 oz	50	69%	4	2.5	1
Gorgonzola crumbles (Athenos), 1 oz	98	69%	8	5	1
Gouda (Boar's Head), 1 oz	110	77%	9	5	2
Gouda, specialty (Sara Lee), 1 oz	109	74%	9	6	0
Jarlsberg, deli style, sliced (Sargento), 1 oz	80	68%	6	3.5	0
Monterey Jack (Boar's Head), 1 oz	105	77%	9	6	0
Monterey Jack (Land-O-Lakes), 1 oz	110	74%	9	6	0
Monterey Jack, reduced fat (Organic Valley), ¼ cup	80	56%	5	3.5	1
Mozzarella, singles, 2% (Kraft), 1 slice	50	60%	2.5	1.5	2
Mozzarella, string, part skim (Organic Valley), 1 oz	81	53%	5	3	1
Mozzarella, part skim, shredded (Organic Valley), ¼ cup	60	58%	5	3	1

Product and Portion Size	Calories	% Cal from Fat	Total Fat (g)	Bad Fat (g)	Net Carbs (g)
Mozzarella, fat free, shredded (Polly-O), 1 oz	40	0%	0	0	1
Mozzarella, part skim (Polly-O), 1 oz	80	56%	5	3.5	1
Mozzarella, deli style, sliced (Sargento), 1 slice	60	60%	4	2.5	1
Muenster, reduced sodium (Alpine Lace), 1 slice	110	72%	9	5	1
Muenster (Boar's Head), 1 oz	100	75%	8	5	0
Muenster (Organic Valley), 1 oz	100	72%	8	5	0
Parmesan, shredded (Organic Valley), ¼ cup	110	61%	7	4	0
Parmesan, grated (Polly-O), 5g	20	75%	1.5	1	0
Parmesan & romano, grated (Polly-O), 5g	20	75%	1.5	1	0
Parmesan, grated (Sargento), 2 tsp	25	63%	1.5	1	0
Provolone, reduced fat and sodium (Alpine Lace), 1 slice	90	63%	6	3.5	1
Provolone (Organic Valley), 1 oz	100	71%	8	5	<1
Ricotta, fat free (Polly-O), ¼ cup	45	0%	0	0	3
Ricotta, part skim (Polly-O), ¼ cup	90	56%	6	4	2
Ricotta, part skim (Sargento), ¼ cup	70	53%	4.5	3	3
Ricotta, whole milk (Sargento), ¼ cup	90	57%	6	4	3
Swiss, baby Swiss (Boar's Head), 1 oz	110	73%	9	6	<1
Swiss, singles 2% (Kraft), 1 slice	50	50%	2.5	1.5	2
Swiss, deli style (Sargento), 1 slice	110	67%	8	4.5	1

Product and Portion Size	Calories	% Cal from Fat	Total Fat (g)	Bad Fat (g)	Net Carbs (g)
CHEESE SUBSTITUTES					
Almond Rella (Rella), 1 oz	70	47%	3.5	0	3
Better Than Cream Cheese, plain (Tofutti), 2 Tbs	80	90%	8	2	1
Better Than Cream Cheese, French onion (Tofutti), 2 Tbs	80	90%	8	2	1
Soy American (Tofutti), 1 slice	70	74%	5	2	2
Soy American (Smart Beat), 1 slice	25	0%	0	0	3
Soy cheddar, Good slice (Yves), 1 slice	36	48%	2	0	1
Soy cheddar, Veggie Shreds (Galaxy), 1.1 oz	59	46%	3	0	2
Soy mozzarella, slices (Tofutti), 1 slice	70	74%	5	3	2
Soy parmesan, mozzarella, romano shreds (Galaxy), 1.1 oz	59	46%	3	0	2
Soy Swiss, Good Slice (Yves), 1 slice	35	47%	2	0	1
Tofu Rella (Rella), 1 oz	80	56%	5	1	3
Vegan Rella (Rella), 1 oz	71	38%	3	0	10
CHEESE SPREADS					
Alouette, garlic & herb, 2 Tbs	60	87%	6	4	1
Alouette, spinach Florentine, 2 Tbs	60	87%	6	3.5	1
Alouette, vegetable garden, 2 Tbs	60	87%	6	4	1
Kraft, bacon, 2 Tbs	90	78%	8	5	1

Product and Portion Size	Calories	% Cal from Fat	Total Fat (g)	Bad Fat (g)	Net Carbs (g)
Kraft, Cheese Whiz, light, 2 Tbs	80	38%	3.5	2	6
Kraft, Cheese Whiz, original, 2 Tbs	90	67%	6	4.5	4
Kraft, Cheese Whiz, salsa con queso, 2 Tbs	90	67%	7	4.5	4
Kraft, Pimento & olive spread, 2 Tbs	80	73%	6	4	3
Kraft, Roca blue, 2 Tbs	80	75%	7	4.5	2
Kraft, Sharp cheese Squeez-A-Snack, 2 Tbs	90	80%	8	5	0
Velveeta, light, 2 Tbs	60	42%	3	2	4
Velveeta, Mexican mild, 2 Tbs	90	69%	6	4	3
Velveeta, original, 2 Tbs	80	63%	6	4	3
CHERRIES					
Raw, sour, red, pitted, 1 cup	77	5%	0	0	19
Raw, sweet, red, pitted, 1 cup	91	2%	9	9	23
Del Monte canned, dark sweet, ½ cup	100	0%	0	0	24
Dole, frozen, 1 cup	90	0%	0	0	19
S&W, dark & sweet, ½ cup	140	0%	0	0	33
CHERRY BEVERAGES					
Hi-C wild cherry, 200 ml drink box	100	0%	0	0	28
Knudsen, black cherry spritzer, 12 oz	180	0%	0	0	46

Product and Portion Size	Calories	% Cal from Fat	Total Fat (g)	Bad Fat (g)	Net Carbs (g)
Knudsen, cherry cider, 8 oz	130	0%	0	0	33
Knudsen, Just black cherry, 8 oz	180	0%	0	0	44
Knudsen, Just tart cherry, organic, 8 oz	130	0%	0	0	32
Kool-Aid, 8 oz	80	0%	0	0	20
Minute Maid Cooler, clear cherry, 200 ml pouch	100	0%	0	0	28
CHESTNUTS					
Chinese, roasted, 1 oz	68	4%	0	0	15
European, roasted, 1 oz	69	7%	0	0	15
Japanese, roasted, 1 oz	57	4%	0	0	13
CHICKEN, canned, Swanson chicken ala king, 10.5 oz	210	52%	12	3.5	12
Swanson chicken breast in water, 2 oz	50	20%	1	0.5	1
CHICKEN, fresh, boiler or fryer					
Breast & skin, roasted, 4 oz	224	36%	8	4	0
Breast only, roasted, 4 oz	188	19%	4	0	0
Dark & skin, roasted, 4 oz	284	56%	16	4	0
Dark only, roasted, 4 oz	232	43%	12	4	0
Drumstick, no skin, fried, 1	82	38%	3	1	0
Leg, no skin, fried, 1	196	40%	9	2	0

Product and Portion Size	Calories	% Cal from Fat	Total Fat (g)	Bad Fat (g)	Net Carbs (g)
Light meat, no skin, fried, 1 cup	269	26%	8	2	1
Thigh, no skin, fried, 1	113	42%	5	1	1
CHICKEN, other					
Capon, meat & skin, roasted, 4 oz	260	46%	12	4	0
Cornish game hen, roasted, 1 bird	245	26%	9	2	0
Giblets, simmered, 1 cup	281	43%	13	4	0
Liver, simmered, 4 oz	188	36%	8	4	0
CHICKEN, refrigerated or frozen					
Organic Valley, ground, frozen, 4 oz	200	55%	12	3	1
Organic Valley, breast, boneless, skinless, 4 oz	120	11%	1.5	0	0
Perdue, breast nuggets, cooked, 5 nuggets	248	55%	16	3.5	15
Perdue, breast tenderloins, skinless, boneless, 3 oz	101	9%	1	0.5	0
Perdue, Cornish hens, cooked, 3 oz	210	60%	14	4.5	0
Tyson					
Breast fillet, 1 pc	240	34%	9	1.5	20
Breast fillet, mesquite, 1 pc	130	47%	7	2	1
Breast, diced strips, 3 oz	68	10%	1	0	0
Chicken Bites, 3 oz	270	60%	18	4	15

Product and Portion Size	Calories	% Cal from Fat	Total Fat (g)	Bad Fat (g)	Net Carbs (g)
Nuggets, frozen, 5 pcs	280	57%	18	4	16
Strips, buffalo style, 2 pcs	230	39%	10	2	29
Strips, crispy chicken, 2 pcs	200	44%	10	2	13
Tenders, honey battered, 5 pcs	220	53%	13	3	13
Wings, hot 'n spicy, 3 pcs	219	62%	15	3.5	1
Weaver					
Breast strips, 3 pcs	230	52%	14	3.5	14
Breast tenders, 5 pcs	240	54%	14	3	15
Buffalo popcorn chicken, 7 pcs	230	52%	14	2	13
Crispy mini-drums, 5 pcs	250	56%	16	3.5	14
Italian style patties, 1	210	57%	14	3	12
Nuggets, 4 nuggets	230	52%	14	3.5	14
Original patties, 1	180	56%	11	2.5	10
CHICKEN SUBSTITUTES					
Morningstar					
Buffalo wings, 5 wings	200	40%	9	1.5	18
Chik 'n Nuggets, 4 nuggets	170	37%	7	1	18
Chik 'n Patties, 1	160	31%	6	1	15
Chik 'n Tenders, 2 pcs	190	32%	7	1	20

Product and Portion Size	Calories	% Cal from Fat	Total Fat (g)	Bad Fat (g)	Net Carbs (g)
Worthington					
Chik Sticks, 6 pcs	100	50%	6	1	4
Diced Chik, fat free, ¼ cup	30	0%	0	0	2
Fried Chik 'n gravy, 2 pcs	150	60%	10	1.5	5
Meatless Chicken roll, ⅜" slice	90	44%	4.5	0.5	2
Meatless Chicken slices, 3 slices	90	50%	4.5	1	2
CHICKPEAS (Garbanzo Beans)					
Eden, organic, ½ cup	130	7%	1	0	23
Progresso, ½ cup	100	15%	1.5	0	17
S&W, ½ cup	80	13%	1	0	19
CHILIS, green, canned					
Pace, diced, 2 Tbs	10	0%	0	0	1
Old El Paso, whole, 1 chile	10	0%	0	0	2
CHILI & CHILI BEANS					
Eden organic chili beans w/jalapeno & red pepper, ½ cup	130	0%	0	0	14
Campbell's Chunky, Firehouse, 1 cup	220	32%	8	3.5	16
Campbell's Chunky, Roadhouse, 1 cup	220	32%	8	3.5	16
Campbell's Sizzling Steak, 1 cup	200	15%	3.5	1.5	22
Fantastic Foods, vegetarian chili, 1 cup	200	8%	2	0	25

Product and Portion Size	Calories	% Cal from Fat	Total Fat (g)	Bad Fat (g)	Net Carbs (g)
Health Valley, 99% f-f vegetarian spicy black bean, 1 cup	160	6%	1	0	17
Health Valley, 99% f-f medium turkey chili, 1 cup	220	11%	3	1	8
Health Valley, mild vegetarian chili, 1 cup	160	6%	1	0	19
Health Valley, vegetarian lentil chili, 1 cup	160	6%	1	0	17
S&W, chili beans, Santa Fe, ½ cup	90	0%	0	0	15
S&W, chili beans, tomato sauce, ½ cup	110	9%	1	0	17
Stagg, Classic Chili, 1 cup	330	45%	17	8	23
Stagg, Country Brand, 1 cup	320	44%	16	7	24
Stagg, Laredo, 1 cup	320	44%	15	7	21
Stagg, Ranch House chicken chili, 1 cup	290	28%	9	3	26
Stagg, Turkey Ranchero, 1 cup	240	10%	3	1	16
Stagg, vegetable Garden 4-bean, 1 cup	200	5%	1	0	30
CHOCOLATE, baking					
Baker's baking unsweetened squares ½ oz	70	86%	7	4.5	2
Baker's bittersweet squares, ½ oz	70	71%	6	3	6
Baker's chocolate chunks semi-sweet, ½ oz	70	57%	4.5	2.5	8
Baker's German sweet, ½ oz	60	50%	3.5	2	7
Baker's Premium white squares, ½ oz	80	50%	4.5	3	8

Product and Portion Size	Calories	% Cal from Fat	Total Fat (g)	Bad Fat (g)	Net Carbs (g)
CLAMS					
Bumble Bee, canned, ¼ cup	50	20%	1	0.5	2
Chicken of the Sea, chopped, ¼ cup	30	0%	0	0	2
Chicken of the Sea, whole baby, ¼ cup	30	0%	0	0	1
Mrs. Paul's fried clams, 3 oz	270	44%	13	2.5	28
COCONUT					
Fresh, raw, shredded, 1 cup	283	79%	27	24	5
Baker's Angel Flake, shredded, sweetened, 2 oz	70	71%	5	4.5	5
Milk, organic lite (Thai Kitchen), 2 oz	45	87%	3	3	1
COD					
Atlantic, baked, 3 oz	**89**	**8%**	**1**	**0**	**0**
Atlantic, canned, 3 oz	**89**	**8%**	**1**	**0**	**0**
Pacific, baked, 3 oz	**88**	**7%**	**1**	**0**	**0**
COFFEE, flavored, General Foods Intl					
Café Francais, 1 serv.	60	42%	3	2.5	8
Crème caramel, 1 serv.	60	25%	2	1.5	12
French vanilla, 1 serv.	60	42%	2.5	0.5	10
French vanilla, sugar free, 1 serv.	30	6%	2.5	2	2

Product and Portion Size	Calories	% Cal from Fat	Total Fat (g)	Bad Fat (g)	Net Carbs (g)
French vanilla nut, 1 serv.	60	42%	2.5	2.5	10
Italian cappucino, 1 serv.	50	30%	1.5	1.5	10
Suisse mocha, 1 serv.	60	25%	2	1.5	10
Viennese chocolate, 1 serv.	50	20%	1.5	1.5	11
COLLARDS, fresh, cooked, no salt, 1 cup	**49**	**12%**	**1**	**0**	**4**
COOKIES, mixes and unbaked					
Betty Crocker					
Chocolate Chip, pouch, 2 cookies	120	25%	3	1.5	21
Chocolate Peanut Butter Chip, pouch, 2 cookies	120	25%	3.5	2.5	19
Oatmeal, pouch, 2 cookies	110	9%	1.5	0	21
Peanut Butter, pouch, 2 cookies	120	29%	4	1	22
Sugar, pouch, 2 cookies	120	21%	2.5	0.5	22
Pillsbury					
Big Deluxe Classic, Chocolate Peanut, 1 cookie	200	45%	10	5.5	24
Big Deluxe Classic, Peanut Butter Cup, 1 cookie	190	42%	9	5	23
Big Deluxe Classic, Turtle Supreme, 1 cookie	200	45%	10	5	24
Chocolate Chip, bake 1 oz	130	46%	7	3.5	16
Chocolate Chip Walnut, 1 cookie	120	50%	7	3	13

Product and Portion Size	Calories	% Cal from Fat	Total Fat (g)	Bad Fat (g)	Net Carbs (g)
Oatmeal Chocolate Chip, 1 oz	130	38%	6	3	16
Ready to Bake Chocolate Candy, 1 cookie	120	42%	5	3	15
Ready to Bake Chocolate Chunk & Chip, 1 cookie	120	42%	6	3	15
Ready to Bake, Sugar, 1 cookie	120	42%	6	3	15
COOKIES, ready-to-eat					
Archway, Double Fudge Crème, 2 cookies	190	42%	9	5.5	25
Archway, Fig bars, 2 cookies	110	16%	2	0	22
Barbara's					
Animal cookies, 8	120	33%	4.5	2.5	17
Chocolate chip, 1	80	44%	4	2	8
Fig bar, apple cinnamon, 1	60	0%	0	0	13
Fig bar, blueberry, 1	70	7%	0.5	0	15
Fig bar, raspberry, 1	60	0%	0	0	13
Fig bar, traditional, 1	60	8%	0.5	0	14
Fig bar, wheat free, 1	60	0%	0	0	12
Fig bar, whole wheat, 1	60	0%	0	0	12
Double Dutch chocolate, 1	80	44%	4	2.5	8
Old-fashioned oatmeal, 1	70	36%	3	1.5	10

Product and Portion Size	Calories	% Cal from Fat	Total Fat (g)	Bad Fat (g)	Net Carbs (g)
Snackimals, chocolate chip, 10 cookies	120	29%	4	0	19
Snackimals, vanilla, 10 cookies	110	32%	4	0	17
Snackimals, wheat free, 10 cookies	120	38%	5	0	16
Traditional shortbread, 1	80	44%	4	3	8
Famous Amos					
Chocolate chip & pecans, 4 cookies	150	47%	8	4	17
Chocolate Crème sandwich, 3 cookies	160	31%	6	4	24
Iced Gingersnaps, low fat, 2 oz pkg	200	12%	3	1.5	39
Oatmeal Chocolate Chip walnut, 4 cookies	140	43%	7	4	17
Oatmeal Raisin, 4 cookies	140	36%	6	4	19
Vanilla Crème sandwich, 3 cookies	170	35%	7	4	25
Health Valley					
Apricot delight, f-f, 3 cookies	100	0%	0	0	21
Café Creations chocolate chip, 1 cookie	100	45%	5	2	11
Chocolate chip oatmeal, 1 cookie	100	35%	4	0.5	13
Chocolate vanilla cream cookie bar, 1	200	35%	8	2.5	31
Cookie crème chocolate sandwich, 2 cookies	120	38%	5	1	19
Oatmeal raisin, 1 cookie	90	30%	3.5	0	13
White chocolate chunk, 1 cookie	140	50%	7	3	17

Product and Portion Size	Calories	% Cal from Fat	Total Fat (g)	Bad Fat (g)	Net Carbs (g)
Keebler					
Animal cookies, frosted, 8 cookies	150	40%	7	6	21
Chip Deluxe, chocolate lovers, 1	80	50%	4.5	3	9
Chips Deluxe, coconut, 1	80	50%	4.5	3.5	8
Chips Deluxe, peanut butter cups, 1	90	44%	4.5	3.5	9
EL Fudge double stuffed, 2 cookies	180	44%	9	5.5	22
Fudge Shoppe, deluxe graham, 3 cookies	140	43%	7	6	16
Fudge Shoppe, filled peanut butter, 2 cookies	170	59%	17	5.5	14
Fudge Shoppe, fudge sticks, 3 cookies	150	47%	8	6.5	19
Fudge Shoppe, reduced fat, fudge stripes, 3 cookies	130	35%	5	4	20
Golden Vanilla wafers, 8 cookies	140	36%	6	3.5	20
Oatmeal, country style, 2 cookies	130	38%	6	4	17
Sandies, chocolate chip pecan, 1 cookie	80	56%	5	2.5	9
Sandies, fruit delights, strawberry cheesecake, 1 cookie	80	38%	3.5	2	11
Sandies, pecan, 1 cookie	80	56%	5	3	9
Sandies, pecan, reduced fat, 1 cookie	80	38%	3.5	2	11
Sandies, simply shortbread, 1 cookie	80	50%	4.5	3	10
Sandies, swirl cinnamon, 1 cookie	90	50%	5	3	9

Product and Portion Size	Calories	% Cal from Fat	Total Fat (g)	Bad Fat (g)	Net Carbs (g)
Soft Batch, chocolate chip, 1 cookie	80	44%	3.5	2	10
Soft Batch, oatmeal raisin, 1 cookie	80	31%	3	1.5	10
Vienna Fingers, 2 cookies	150	40%	7	4	21
Vienna Fingers, reduced fat, 2 cookies	140	32%	5	3	23
Murray Sugar Free					
Chocolate chip, 3 cookies	140	50%	8	5	20
Chocolate sandwich cream, 3 cookies	130	46%	7	4	17
Double fudge, 3 cookies	140	43%	7	4	21
Lemon wafers, 4 cookies	130	54%	8	4.5	15
Oatmeal, 3 cookies	150	40%	7	4	19
Peanut butter, 3 cookies	140	57%	9	4	15
Shortbread, 8 cookies	140	38%	6	3.5	20
Shortbread, pecan, 3 cookies	170	59%	11	6	17
Vanilla wafers, 9	130	35%	5	3.5	23
Nabisco					
Chips Ahoy, 100% whole grain, 1 cookie	150	47%	8	2.5	20
Chips Ahoy, Chocolate Chip, 33g	160	44%	8	2.5	21
Chips Ahoy, Chunky Chocolate Chip, 16g	80	44%	4	1.5	9

Product and Portion Size	Calories	% Cal from Fat	Total Fat (g)	Bad Fat (g)	Net Carbs (g)
Chips Ahoy, Chunky White Fudge, 1 cookie	80	50%	4.5	1.5	9
Chips Ahoy, Reduced Fat, 1 cookie	140	36%	5	2	22
Chips Ahoy, Soft Baked Chunky, 1 cookie	120	38%	5	2.5	18
Fig Newtons, 100% whole grain, 2 cookies	110	18%	2	0.5	20
Fig Newtons, f-f, 2 cookies	90	0%	0	0	21
Fig Newtons, original, 2 cookies	110	18%	2	0	21
Nilla Wafers, original, 1 oz	140	36%	6	1.5	21
Nilla Wafers, reduced fat, 1 oz	120	17%	2	0	24
Nutter Butter sandwich, 2 cookies	130	38%	5	1.5	18
Oreo sandwich, 3 cookies	160	38%	7	2	24
Oreo sandwich, Chocolate Crème, 2 cookies	150	40%	7	2.5	20
Oreo sandwich, Double Stuf, 2 cookies	140	43%	7	2.5	19
Oreo sandwich, reduced fat, 3 cookies	150	27%	4.5	1	25
Snackwells, crème sandwich, 2 cookies	110	23%	3	0.5	20
Snackwells, Devil's food, f-f, 1 cookie	50	0%	0	0	12
Pepperidge Farm					
Bordeaux, 4 cookies	130	38%	5	3.5	18
Brussels, 3 cookies	150	42%	7	4	19

Product and Portion Size	Calories	% Cal from Fat	Total Fat (g)	Bad Fat (g)	Net Carbs (g)
Chocolate Chunk milk chocolate macadamia, 1 cookie	140	50%	8	3.5	16
Chocolate Chunk white chocolate macadamia, 1 cookie	130	42%	6	4	16
Double Chocolate Chunk, dark chocolate, 1 cookie	140	45%	7	3	17
Geneva, 3 cookies	160	51%	9	4	18
Gingerbread Man, 4 cookies	130	27%	4	2	20
Milano Double Chocolate, 2 cookies	140	50%	8	4	16
Milano, original 3 cookies	180	50%	10	5	20
Shortbread, 2 cookies	140	50%	7	4	15
Soft Bake, Chocolate Chunk, 1 cookie	150	47%	8	3.5	20
Soft Bake, Snickerdoodle, 1 cookie	140	32%	5	2.5	21
Soft Bake, sugar, 1 cookie	140	32%	5	2.5	22
Sugar, 3 cookies	140	43%	6	2.5	19
Verona Strawberry, 3 cookies	140	32%	5	2.5	21
CORN					
Fresh, cooked, white or yellow, no salt, 1 cup	177	10%	2	0	24
Fresh, cooked, white or yellow, cob, 7"	111	10%	1	0	23
Canned					
Del Monte, Savory Sides, in butter sauce, ½ cup	90	28%	2.5	1	13

Product and Portion Size	Calories	% Cal from Fat	Total Fat (g)	Bad Fat (g)	Net Carbs (g)
Del Monte, Savory Sides, Fiesta corn, ½ cup	50	10%	1	0	10
Del Monte, Savory Sides, gold & white, ½ cup	80	6%	0.5	0	16
Del Monte, Savory Sides, Santa Fe, ½ cup	70	7%	1	0	15
Del Monte, Savory Sides, white, cream, ½ cup	100	10%	1	0	19
Del Monte, Savory Sides, whole kernel, ½ cup	90	11%	1	0	15
Green Giant, creamed corn, ½ cup	90	6%	0.5	0	18
Green Giant, extra sweet niblets, ⅓ cup	50	10%	0.5	0	9
Green Giant, Mexicorn, ⅓ cup	70	7%	0.5	0	13
Green Giant, whole kernel sweet, ½ cup	80	6%	0.5	0	16
S&W, creamed corn, ½ cup	60	8%	0.5	0	12
S&W, whole kernels, ½ cup	60	17%	1	0	8
Frozen					
Birds Eye, baby gold & white, ⅔ cup	100	9%	1	0	18
Birds Eye, baby white corn kernels, ⅔ cup	90	10%	1	0	15
Birds Eye, baby corn & vegetable blend, ¾ cup	70	0%	0	0	11
Birds Eye, super sweet kernel corn, ⅔ cup	70	13%	1	0	12
Birds Eye, sweet corn & bacon in cheese sauce, ½ cup	150	24%	4	1.5	25
Birds Eye, sweet corn & butter sauce, ½ cup	150	18%	3	1	26

Product and Portion Size	Calories	% Cal from Fat	Total Fat (g)	Bad Fat (g)	Net Carbs (g)
Birds Eye, sweet kernel corn, ⅔ cup	100	9%	1	0	20
Cascadian Farms, organic sweet corn, ¾ cup	70	7%	0.5	0	16
C&W, salsa corn, 1 cup	90	6%	0.5	0	14
Green Giant, cob, niblets, 1 ear	150	7%	1	0	29
Green Giant, cream style, ½ cup	110	9%	1	0	21
Green Giant, niblets w/butter, ⅔ cup	110	14%	1.5	0.5	20
Green Giant, shoepeg white corn, no sauce, ½ cup	70	14%	1	0	13
CORN CHIPS					
Bugles, chili cheese, 1⅓ cup	160	50%	9	7	18
Bugles, original, 1⅓ cup	160	50%	9	8	17
Bugles, salsa, 1⅓ cup	160	50%	9	7	18
Bugles, Smokin' BBQ, 1⅓ cup	150	47%	8	7	18
Bugles, SW ranch, 1⅓ cup	170	53%	10	1.5	18
Doritos, Cool ranch tortilla, 1 oz	140	43%	7	1	17
Doritos, Cool ranch tortilla, baked, 1 oz	120	25%	3.5	0.5	19
Doritos, Light nacho cheese, 1 oz	100	20%	2	0.5	17
Doritos, Nacho cheese tortilla, 1 oz	140	50%	8	1.5	16
Doritos, Nacho cheese tortilla, baked, 1 oz	120	25%	3.5	0.5	19

Product and Portion Size	Calories	% Cal from Fat	Total Fat (g)	Bad Fat (g)	Net Carbs (g)
Doritos, Ranchero tortilla, 1 oz	150	47%	8	1	16
Doritos, Rollitos cooler ranch, 1 oz	140	50%	8	1.5	16
Doritos, Rollitos nacho cheesier, 1 oz	150	47%	8	1.5	16
Doritos, Rollitos, zesty taco, 1 oz	150	47%	8	1.5	16
Doritos, Spicy nacho, 1 oz	140	43%	7	1	17
Doritos, Toasted corn, 1 oz	140	43%	7	1	17
Fritos, bar-b-q, 1 oz	150	60%	10	1.5	15
Fritos, cheese flavor, 1 oz	160	56%	10	1.5	14
Fritos, king size, 1 oz	160	56%	10	1.5	15
Fritos, flamin' hot, 1 oz	160	56%	10	1.5	14
Fritos, king size, 1 oz	160	56%	10	1.5	15
Fritos, original, 1 oz	160	56%	10	1.5	14
Fritos, Scoops, 1 oz	160	56%	10	1.5	15
Herr's, bite size dippers, 1 oz	140	36%	6	1.5	16
Herr's, corn chips, 1 oz	160	56%	10	2	15
Herr's, Mexican cheddar dippers, 1 oz	150	43%	7	2	16
Herr's, Nachitos, 1 oz	140	36%	6	1	16
Tostitos, natural blue corn, 1 oz	140	36%	6	0.5	18

Product and Portion Size	Calories	% Cal from Fat	Total Fat (g)	Bad Fat (g)	Net Carbs (g)
Tostitos, original bite size, baked, 1 oz	110	5%	1	0	22
Tostitos, restaurant style tortilla, 1 oz	140	43%	7	1	18
Tostitos, Santa Fe rounds, 1 oz	140	36%	6	0.5	18
Tostitos, Sensations red chile & lime, 1 oz	150	47%	8	1.5	15
Tostitos, Sensations southwestern ranch, 1 oz	150	47%	8	1.5	16
Wise, Dipsy Doodles, rippled, 1 oz	160	56%	10	2.5	15
Wise, Nacho Twister, 1 oz	160	63%	11	3	13
COUSCOUS					
Fantastic Foods					
Organic, ¼ cup prep.	150	3%	0.5	0	32
Organic, whole wheat, ¼ cup uncooked	170	3%	0.5	0	31
Near East					
Herb Chicken, 2 oz mix	190	5%	1	0	37
Mediterranean Curry, 2 oz mix	190	5%	1	0	37
Original plain, ⅓ cup dry	220	5%	1	0	44
Parmesan, 2 oz mix	200	10%	2	0.5	37
Toasted Pine Nut, 2 oz mix	200	13%	3	0.5	36
Tomato Lentil, 2 oz mix	190	5%	1	0	37

Product and Portion Size	Calories	% Cal from Fat	Total Fat (g)	Bad Fat (g)	Net Carbs (g)
CRAB					
Bumble Bee, canned, white, ¼ cup	40	25%	1	0	0
Chicken of the Sea, canned, fancy, 2 oz	40	0%	0	0	2
Fresh, cooked, blue, 1 cup	120	17%	2	0	0
Fresh, cooked, Dungeness, 3 oz	93	11%	1	0	1
CRACKERS					
Eden Foods, brown rice, 8 crackers	120	13%	2	0	20
Eden Foods, nori maki rice, 15 crackers	110	0%	0	0	22
Health Valley					
Bruschetta Vegetable, no salt added, 6	60	25%	1.5	0	9
Butter corn bread crackers, 4	60	25%	1.5	0	10
Garden herb, low fat, 5 crackers	60	25%	1.5	0	9
Honey corn bread crackers, 4	60	25%	1.5	0	10
Original oat bran graham, 6	120	21%	3	0	19
Sesame, low fat, 5	60	25%	1.5	0	9
Stoned wheat, low fat, 5	60	17%	1	0	9
Keebler					
Club, original, 4 crackers	70	36%	3	1	8

Product and Portion Size	Calories	% Cal from Fat	Total Fat (g)	Bad Fat (g)	Net Carbs (g)
Club, reduced fat, 5 crackers	70	29%	2.5	0.5	11
Grahams, cinnamon crisp, 8	130	23%	3.5	1	22
Grahams, cinnamon crisp, low fat, 8	110	14%	1.5	0	22
Grahams, honey, 8	140	25%	4	1	22
Grahams, original, 8	130	23%	3.5	1	21
Scooby-Doo graham cracker sticks, 9	130	27%	4	0.5	20
Scooby-Doo graham cracker sticks, honey, 9	130	27%	4	0.5	20
Sunshine, Cheez-It, cheddar jack, 25 crackers	160	44%	8	2.5	18
Sunshine, Cheez-It, Fiesta cheddar nacho, 25 crackers	160	44%	8	2.5	17
Sunshine, Cheez-It, hot & spicy, 25 crackers	150	47%	8	2	17
Sunshine, Cheez-It, original, 27 crackers	160	44%	8	2	17
Sunshine, Cheez-It, reduced fat, 29 crackers	130	31%	4	1	19
Sunshine, Cheez-It, Twisterz, cool ranch, 17 crackers	140	36%	6	2.5	19
Sunshine, Cheez-It, Twisterz, hot wings cheesy blue, 17	140	36%	6	2.5	18
Sunshine, Cheez-It, white cheddar, 25 crackers	150	47%	8	2.5	17
Sunshine Krispy, original, 5 crackers	60	25%	1.5	1	10
Sunshine, Krispy, soup & oyster, 5	70	21%	1.5	0.5	12
Sunshine, Krispy, whole wheat, 5	60	25%	1.5	1	10

Product and Portion Size	Calories	% Cal from Fat	Total Fat (g)	Bad Fat (g)	Net Carbs (g)
Toasteds, Buttercrisp, 5	80	38%	3.5	1	9
Toasteds, Onion, 5	80	38%	3.5	1	10
Toasteds, Sesame, 5	80	38%	3.5	1	9
Toasteds, Wheat, 5	80	38%	3.5	2	9
Townhouse Bistro, corn bread, 2 crackers	80	31%	3	1.5	10
Townhouse Bistro, low salt, 5	80	50%	4.5	1	9
Townhouse Bistro, multigrain, 2	80	31%	3	1.5	10
Townhouse Bistro, original, 5	80	50%	4.5	1	8
Townhouse Bistro, reduced fat, 6 crackers	60	25%	1.5	0.5	10
Townhouse Bistro, rye 2 crackers	70	36%	3	1.5	10
Townhouse Bistro, wheat, 5 crackers	80	44%	4	1	9
Wheatables, 7 grain, 17 crackers	140	36%	6	1.5	19
Wheatables, honey wheat, 17 crackers	140	36%	6	1.5	19
Wheatables, original, 17 crackers	140	36%	6	1.5	19
Wheatables, reduced fat, 19 crackers	140	25%	4	1	22
Zesta, f-f, 5 crackers	60	0%	0	0	12
Zesta, original, 5 crackers	60	25%	1.5	1	10
Zesta, whole grain wheat, 5 crackers	60	25%	1.5	1	10

Product and Portion Size	Calories	% Cal from Fat	Total Fat (g)	Bad Fat (g)	Net Carbs (g)
Nabisco					
Cheese Nips, cheddar, 1 oz	150	40%	7	1.5	17
Cheese Nips, four cheese, 1 oz	150	40%	7	1.5	17
Ritz Bits, cracker sandwich, peanut butter, 1 oz	140	50%	8	1.5	15
Ritz, Dinosaurs, 1 oz	130	27%	4	1	21
Ritz, original, ½ oz	80	44%	4	1	10
Ritz, reduced fat, ½ oz	70	21%	2	0	11
Ritz, Top-ems, ½ oz	70	36%	3	0.5	10
Ritz, whole wheat, ½ oz	70	29%	2.5	0.5	10
Triscuit, deli-style rye, 1 oz	120	30%	4.5	0.5	16
Triscuit, garden herb, 1 oz	120	29%	4	0.5	17
Triscuit, original, 1 oz	120	30%	4.5	0.5	16
Triscuit, reduced fat, 1 oz	120	21%	3	0	18
Wheat Thins, honey, 1 oz	150	30%	6	1	20
Wheat Thins, multigrain, 1 oz	130	31%	4.5	0.5	20
Wheat Thins, original, 1 oz	150	30%	6	1	20
Wheat Thins, ranch, 1 oz	140	43%	6	1	18
Wheat Thins, reduced fat, 1 oz	130	27%	4	0.5	20

Product and Portion Size	Calories	% Cal from Fat	Total Fat (g)	Bad Fat (g)	Net Carbs (g)
Old London					
Melba Flatbread crackers, sesame, 2 crackers	60	30%	2	0	8
Melba JJ Flats, Flavorall, 1 cracker	60	37%	2.5	0.5	8
Melba JJ Flats, sesame, 1 cracker	60	30%	2	0	8
Melba rounds (12-grain, vegetable), 5 crackers	50	0%	0	0	11
Melba Snacks (onion), 5 crackers	60	20%	1.5	0	11
Melba Toast (white, garlic, or wheat), 3 pcs	50	0%	0	0	10
Pepperidge Farm Goldfish					
Baby, 89 pcs	140	32%	5	1	19
Cheddar, 55 pcs	140	32%	5	1	19
Original, 55 pcs	150	37%	6	0.5	19
Parmesan, 60 pcs	130	27%	4	1	19
Pizza, 55 pcs	140	32%	5	1	19
Pretzel, 43 pcs	130	18%	2.5	0.5	23
CRANBERRY					
Dried, sweetened (S&W Craisins), ⅓ cup	130	0%	0	0	31
Fresh, raw, 1 cup	51	2%	0	0	8
Sauce, canned, whole berry (S&W), ¼ cup	100	0%	0	0	25

Product and Portion Size	Calories	% Cal from Fat	Total Fat (g)	Bad Fat (g)	Net Carbs (g)
Sauce, canned, jellied (S&W), ¼ cup	100	0%	0	0	26
CRANBERRY BEVERAGES					
Langers, cranberry juice cocktail, 8 oz	140	0%	0	0	35
Langers, diet cranberry, 8 oz	30	0%	0	0	8
Langers, white cranberry, 8 oz	120	0%	0	0	28
Langers, white cranberry raspberry, 8 oz	120	0%	0	0	28
Ocean Spray, 100% cocktail, 8 oz	130	0%	0	0	33
Ocean Spray, Cran-Apple, 8 oz	140	0%	0	0	35
Santa Cruz, cranberry nectar, organic, 8 oz	110	0%	0	0	27
CREAM					
Half & half, 1 oz	39	77%	3	2	1
Half & half, f-f, 1 oz	18	21%	0	0	3
Heavy whipping cream, 1 oz	103	94%	11	7	1
Light whipping cream, 1 oz	83	93%	9	5	1
CREAMERS (COFFEE)					
Coffee-Mate, liquid, Amaretto, 1 Tbs	35	43%	1.5	0	5
Coffee-Mate, liquid, chocolate raspberry, 1 Tbs	35	43%	1.5	0	5
Coffee-Mate, liquid, cinnamon vanilla crème, 1 Tbs	35	43%	1.5	0	5

Product and Portion Size	Calories	% Cal from Fat	Total Fat (g)	Bad Fat (g)	Net Carbs (g)
Coffee-Mate, liquid, French vanilla, f-f, 1 Tbs	25	0%	0	0	5
Coffee-Mate Latte Creations, half & half vanilla, 1 Tbs	60	58%	4	2.5	7
Coffee-Mate, powder, coconut crème, 4 tsp	60	42%	3	3	8
Coffee-Mate, powder, creamy chocolate, 4 tsp	60	42%	2.5	2	9
Coffee-Mate, powder, vanilla caramel, 4 tsp	60	42%	3	2.5	9
International Delight, Amaretto, 1 Tbs	40	38%	1.5	1	7
International Delight, chocolate caramel, 1 Tbs	45	44%	2	1	7
International Delight, French vanilla, 1 Tbs	40	38%	2	1	7
International Delight, Irish crème, f-f, 1 Tbs	30	0%	0	0	7
CROUTONS					
Mrs. Cubbison's garlic & butter, 8 pcs	30	33%	1	0	5
Pepperidge Farm, Classic Caesar, 6 pcs	35	37%	1.5	0	5
Pepperidge Farm, Four cheese & garlic, 6 pcs	30	30%	1	0	5
Pepperidge Farm, Onion & garlic, 6 pcs	30	30%	1	0	5
Pepperidge Farm, Whole grain Caesar, 6 pcs	35	26%	1	0	5
Pepperidge Farm, Zesty Italian, 6 pcs	30	30%	1	0	5
CUCUMBER, raw, sliced, peeled, 1 cup	14	12%	0	0	2
CURRANTS, raw, red & white, 1 cup	63	3%	0	0	10
Zante (Sun-Maid), ¼ cup	120	0%	0	0	28

Product and Portion Size	Calories	% Cal from Fat	Total Fat (g)	Bad Fat (g)	Net Carbs (g)
DANDELION GREENS, cooked, no salt, 1 cup chopped	**35**	**15%**	**1**	**0**	**4**
DATES, pitted, chopped, 1 oz	80	1%	0	0	19
Pitted (Dole), ¼ cup	120	0%	0	0	30
Pitted (Sun-Maid), ¼ cup	110	0%	0	0	26
DESSERT TOPPINGS					
Cool Whip, chocolate 9g	25	100%	1.5	1.5	2
Cool Whip, French vanilla, 9g	25	100%	1.5	1.5	2
Cool Whip, lite, 9g	20	50%	1	1	3
Cool Whip, regular, 9g	25	60%	1.5	1.5	2
Cool Whip, sugar free, 9g	20	50%	1	1	3
Smucker's butterscotch caramel, 2 Tbs	130	8%	1	0.5	29
Smucker's Dove dark chocolate, 2 Tbs	140	32%	5	1.5	21
Smucker's Plate Scrapers caramel, 2 Tbs	100	0%	0	0	25
Smucker's Plate Scrapers raspberry, 2 Tbs	100	0%	0	0	25
Smucker's Plate Scrapers vanilla, 2 Tbs	110	9%	1	0	24
Smucker's special recipe hot fudge, 2 Tbs	140	29%	4	1	21
DIPS					
Kraft, bacon & cheddar, 1 oz	60	75%	5	3.5	3
Kraft, creamy ranch, 1 oz	60	67%	4.5	3	3

Product and Portion Size	Calories	% Cal from Fat	Total Fat (g)	Bad Fat (g)	Net Carbs (g)
Kraft, French onion, 1 oz	60	67%	4.5	3	3
Kraft, green onion, 1 oz	60	67%	4	3	4
Kraft, guacamole, 1 oz	50	80%	4.5	2.5	3
Lay's, creamy ranch, 2 Tbs	60	75%	5	2.5	1
Lay's, French onion, 2 Tbs	50	90%	5	2	1
DOUGHNUTS (also see Fast Food, Dunkin Donuts)					
Entenmann's, cinnamon, 1	240	50%	13	7	27
Entenmann's devil's food, 1	310	55%	19	6	34
Entenmann's devil's food crumb, 1	260	45%	13	7	25
Entenmann's plain, 1	210	56%	13	6	21
Entenmann's powdered, 1	240	50%	13	6	27
Tastykake, cinnamon holes, 4 holes	210	43%	10	2	27
Tastykake, glazed holes, blueberry, 4 holes	220	50%	12	10.5	26
Tastykake, glazed holes, chocolate, 4 holes	220	50%	13	12	25
Tastykake, powdered holes, 4 holes	210	43%	10	5	7
DUCK, roasted w/skin, diced, 1 cup	472	76%	40	14	0
Roasted, without skin, diced, 1 cup	281	50%	16	6	0
EGGS					

Product and Portion Size	Calories	% Cal from Fat	Total Fat (g)	Bad Fat (g)	Net Carbs (g)
Chicken, whole, raw, large, 1	73	61%	5	2	0
Chicken, white only, large, 1	17	3%	0	0	0
Chicken, yolk only, large, 1	55	74%	5	2	1
Chicken, whole, hard boiled, large, 1	77	62%	5	2	1
Chicken, whole, poached, large, 1	73	61%	5	2	0
Duck, whole, fresh, 1	129	67%	10	3	1
Goose, whole, fresh, 1	266	65%	19	5	2
Quail, whole, fresh, 1	14	63%	1	0	0
EGG SUBSTITUTES					
Ener-G-Egg, 1½ tsp	15	0%	0	0	4
Morningstar Better 'n Eggs, ¼ cup	20	0%	0	0	0
Morningstar Scramblers, ¼ cup	35	0%	0	0	2
EGGPLANT, boiled, no salt, 1 cup cubes	3	5%	0	0	9
ENDIVE, raw, 1 cup chopped	8	0%	0	0	2
FAST FOOD—Arby's					
Arby's Melt, 1 sandwich	300	36%	12	5.5	34
Apple turnover, no icing, 1	250	54%	15	10	33
Bacon Biscuit, 1	300	53%	17	5	26

Product and Portion Size	Calories	% Cal from Fat	Total Fat (g)	Bad Fat (g)	Net Carbs (g)
Bacon, Beef & Cheddar sandwich	520	47%	27	11	25
Bacon & Egg Croissant, 1	410	56%	26	12	30
Beef & Cheddar sandwich	440	43%	21	9	42
Buttermilk ranch dressing, 1 packet	290	93%	30	6	2
Chicken breast fillet, crispy, 1	640	47%	33	7	50
Chicken breast fillet, grilled, 1	410	37%	17	3	33
Chicken fingers, 3 pack	430	44%	21	6	30
Chicken fingers, 5 pack	720	44%	35	11	50
Chicken salad sandwich w/pecans, 1	880	47%	46	8	85
Corned beef reuben, 1	610	39%	27	8	52
Cool ranch sour cream dipping, 1 packet	160	88%	16	4	2
Curly fries, small	340	53%	20	6.5	35
Curly fries, medium	410	54%	24	8.5	42
Curly fries, large	630	54%	37	13	66
Gourmet chocolate cookie, 1	200	45%	10	6	25
Honey mustard dipping, 1 packet	130	85%	12	3	5
Hot ham & swiss melt, 1	270	18%	8	3.5	34
Jalapeno bites, regular, 5	310	61%	21	11	3

Product and Portion Size	Calories	% Cal from Fat	Total Fat (g)	Bad Fat (g)	Net Carbs (g)
Jr. roast beef sandwich, 1	270	33%	9	4.5	32
Kid's Meal, 2 Pak chicken tenders	290	45%	14	3.5	20
Loaded potato bites, 5, small	350	57%	22	9	25
Loaded potato bites, 10, large	710	57%	44	17	49
Mozzarella sticks, regular, 4	430	58%	28	15.5	36
Onion petals, regular, 43	330	63%	23	5	33
Roast beef, regular	320	38%	14	6	32
Roast beef, medium	420	45%	21	10	32
Roast beef, large	550	47%	28	14	38
Roast turkey & swiss sandwich	720	35%	30	9	69
Roast turkey, ranch & bacon wrap	700	47%	37	12	39
Salad: Chicken club, no dressing	500	48%	9	7	27
Salad: Martha's Vineyard, no dressing	270	26%	8	4	18
Salad: Santa Fe, no dressing	490	43%	23	10	34
Sausage biscuit, 1	390	64%	27	9	25
Sausage, Egg & Cheese wrap	720	57%	45	16	51
Shakes: vanilla, strawberry, Jamoca, regular	500	24%	13	8	81
Shakes: chocolate, regular	510	24%	13	8	83

Product and Portion Size	Calories	% Cal from Fat	Total Fat (g)	Bad Fat (g)	Net Carbs (g)
Sourdough bacon, egg & swiss sandwich	500	53%	29	10	32
Super roast beef sandwich, 1	400	43%	19	7	39
Tangy southwest sauce, 1 packet	330	94%	35	7	5
Ultimate BLT sandwich	780	53%	45	12	69
FAST FOOD—Baskin Robbins					
Banana nut, ½ cup	260	54%	16	7	26
Black walnut, ½ cup	280	61%	19	9	24
Cherries jubilee, ½ cup	240	46%	12	7	29
Chocolate, ½ cup	260	50%	14	9	33
Chocolate almond, ½ cup	300	57%	18	9	31
Chocolate chip cookie dough, ½ cup	290	48%	15	10	35
Chocolate chip, ½ cup	270	52%	16	10	27
Chocolate fudge, ½ cup	270	52%	15	10	35
Chocolate oreo, ½ cup	330	52%	19	9	38
French vanilla, ½ cup	280	57%	18	11.5	26
Fudge brownie, ½ cup	300	57%	19	11	34
German chocolate cake, ½ cup	300	50%	16	9	35
Jamoca, ½ cup	240	50%	13	9	26

Product and Portion Size	Calories	% Cal from Fat	Total Fat (g)	Bad Fat (g)	Net Carbs (g)
Mint chocolate chip, ½ cup	270	52%	16	10	28
Nutty coconut, ½ cup	300	60%	20	9	28
Old fashioned butter pecan, ½ cup	280	57%	18	9	23
Oreo cookies 'n cream, ½ cup	280	50%	15	9	31
Peanut butter & chocolate, ½ cup	320	56%	20	9	30
Pistachio almond, ½ cup	290	59%	19	9	24
Praline & cream, ½ cup	270	44%	14	8	34
Rocky road, ½ cup	290	48%	15	8	35
Vanilla, ½ cup	260	54%	16	10.5	26
Very berry strawberry, ½ cup	220	45%	11	7	28
Low-Fat, No Sugar Added Ice Cream					
Berries & bananas, ½ cup	110	14%	2	1	24
Blueberry swirl, ½ cup	130	15%	2	1	30
Caramel turtle, ½ cup	160	22%	4	3	37
Chocolate chip, ½ cup	170	24%	4.5	3.5	29
Tin roof sundae, ½ cup	190	16%	3	1.5	33
Sundaes					
2 scoop hot fudge sundae	530	50%	29	19	62

Product and Portion Size	Calories	% Cal from Fat	Total Fat (g)	Bad Fat (g)	Net Carbs (g)
3 scoop hot fudge sundae	750	50%	41	27	86
Banana royale	630	38%	27	16	91
Banana split	1030	34%	39	23	168
Happy camper waffle cone sundae	820	45%	41	18.5	107
Nonfat soft serve yogurt, no sugar added					
Butter pecan, ½ cup	90	0%	0	0	16
Café mocha, ½ cup	90	0%	0	0	17
Chocolate, ½ cup	80	0%	0	0	15
Strawberry patch, ½ cup	90	0%	0	0	16
Vanilla, ½ cup	90	0%	0	0	16
Sherbert					
Blue raspberry, ½ cup	160	13%	2	1.5	34
Rock & pop, ½ cup	190	21%	4	3	37
Twisted chip, ½ cup	180	14%	3	2	36
Wild & reckless spirit, ½ cup	160	13%	2	1.5	33
FAST FOOD—Boston Market					
Meals & Sandwiches					
Beef meatloaf, 7.6 oz	480	63%	33	13	21

Product and Portion Size	Calories	% Cal from Fat	Total Fat (g)	Bad Fat (g)	Net Carbs (g)
Boston chicken carver sandwich, 1	690	42%	32	7	53
Boston sirloin dip carver sandwich, 1	920	42%	43	19	67
Boston turkey carver sandwich, 1	830	39%	36	8	67
Chicken, 3 piece dark, individual meal	390	46%	20	6	3
Chicken, ¼ dark rotisserie, no skin	260	46%	13	4	2
Chicken, ¼ white rotisserie, no skin	250	32%	8	2.5	4
Chicken pot pie, 1	800	55%	49	18	55
Meatloaf carver sandwich, 1	940	43%	45	18	90
Roasted turkey, 5 oz	10	17%	3	1	0
Sides & Desserts					
Apple pie, slice	420	43%	20	9	54
Butternut squash, 1 serv.	140	29%	4.5	3	23
Chicken tortilla soup w/toppings	340	59%	22	7	23
Chocolate cake, slice	600	48%	32	11.5	73
Chocolate chip fudge brownie, 1	580	36%	23	5	78
Chocolate fudge bliss, 1	300	23%	8	6	56
Cinnamon apple, 1	210	12%	3	0	44
Corn, 1 serv.	170	21%	4	1	35

Product and Portion Size	Calories	% Cal from Fat	Total Fat (g)	Bad Fat (g)	Net Carbs (g)
Garlic dill potatoes, 1 serv.	140	21%	3	1	21
Macaroni & cheese, 1 serv.	330	33%	12	7.5	38
Mashed potatoes w/gravy, 1 serv.	235	38%	10	6	29
Spinach w/garlic butter, 1 serv.	130	62%	9	6	4
Strawberry bliss, 1	370	57%	23	10	37
Sweet potato casserole, 1	460	33%	17	6	74
Vegetable stuffing, 1 serv.	190	37%	8	1	23
FAST FOOD—Burger King					
Angus steak burger, 1	560	36%	22	9.5	56
Bacon cheeseburger, 1	370	46%	19	8.5	30
BK Big fish, 1	630	43%	30	8.5	63
BK Big fish, w/o tartar sauce	470	26%	13	5	62
BK Chicken fries, 9 pcs	470	60%	31	10.5	26
BK Veggie burger, 1	420	10%	4.5	2.5	39
Cheeseburger, 1	330	42%	16	7.5	30
Chicken Tenders 8 pcs	340	53%	20	8	20
Croisan'wich w/ham, egg, cheese, 1	340	47%	18	8	25
Double Croissan'wich w/double sausage, 1	680	68%	51	21	25

Product and Portion Size	Calories	% Cal from Fat	Total Fat (g)	Bad Fat (g)	Net Carbs (g)
Double Whopper, 1	900	57%	57	21	48
Double Whopper w/cheese, 1	990	59%	64	26.5	49
Dutch apple pie, 1	300	40%	13	6	44
Enormous omelet sandwich, 1	740	55%	46	18	42
French fries, salted, medium	360	50%	20	9	37
French fries, unsalted, medium	360	50%	20	9	37
French toast sticks, 5	390	46%	20	9	44
Garden salad, side, 1	20	0%	0	0	3
Hamburger, 1	290	38%	12	5	29
Hash browns, 1 serv.	230	56%	15	9	21
Icee cherry, medium	140	0%	0	0	40
Low-carb angus steak burger, 1	260	62%	18	8	1
Minute Maid orange juice, 1	140	0%	0	0	33
Onion rings, medium	320	44%	16	7.5	37
Original chicken sandwich, 1	660	55%	40	10.5	48
Shake, chocolate, medium	690	26%	20	12	112
Shake, strawberry, medium	660	26%	19	12	111
Shake, vanilla, medium	560	34%	21	13.5	79

Product and Portion Size	Calories	% Cal from Fat	Total Fat (g)	Bad Fat (g)	Net Carbs (g)
Tendercrisp chicken sandwich, 1	780	50%	43	12	69
Tendercrisp Caesar salad, 1	400	48%	21	8.5	27
Tendercrisp garden salad, 1	410	46%	21	8.5	62
Tendergrill chicken sandwich, 1	450	20%	10	2	49
Tendergrill garden salad, 1	230	30%	8	3	3
Triple Whopper sandwich, 1	1130	59%	74	30	48
Triple Whopper sandwich w/cheese, 1	1230	60%	82	35.5	49
Whopper sandwich, 1	670	52%	39	12.5	48
Whopper jr. sandwich, 1	370	51%	21	6.5	29
Whopper jr sandwich w/cheese, 1	410	54%	24	9	30
FAST FOOD—Church's Chicken					
Apple pie, 1	260	38%	11	6	38
Cajun rice, regular	130	48%	7	3	15
Chicken fried steak sandwich, 1	490	67%	32	10	36
Chicken fried steak w/gravy, 2 pcs	610	63%	43	17	29
Cole slaw, regular	150	60%	10	2	13
Double lemon pie, 1	300	42%	14	6	39
French fries, reg.	420	43%	20	12	49

Product and Portion Size	Calories	% Cal from Fat	Total Fat (g)	Bad Fat (g)	Net Carbs (g)
Jalapeno bombers, 4	240	38%	10	6	26
Macaroni & cheese, reg	210	47%	11	4	22
Mashed potatoes w/gravy, reg	70	26%	2	0	11
Okra, reg.	300	69%	23	4	21
Original breast, 1	200	33%	11	5	2
Original leg, 1	110	49%	6	3	3
Original tender strip, 1 pc	120	45%	6	3	5
Original thigh, 1	330	63%	23	9	7
Original wing, 1	300	57%	19	8	4
Spicy chicken sandwich, 1	360	45%	18	5.5	32
Spicy fish sandwich, 1	320	56%	20	7	23
Spicy popcorn chicken, reg	430	48%	23	6	31
Spicy tender strips, 1 pc	135	47%	7	4	3
Strawberry cream cheese pie, 1 pie	280	48%	15	8	30
FAST FOOD—Dairy Queen					
Desserts, Beverages					
Blizzard, banana split, small	460	28%	14	9	72
Blizzard, banana split, medium	580	26%	17	11.5	96

Product and Portion Size	Calories	% Cal from Fat	Total Fat (g)	Bad Fat (g)	Net Carbs (g)
Blizzard, banana split, large	810	26%	23	16	132
Blizzard, chocolate chip cookie dough, small	720	35%	28	16.5	105
Blizzard, chocolate chip cookie dough, medium	1030	35%	40	24	150
Blizzard, chocolate chip cookie dough, large	1320	35%	52	31	193
Blizzard, Oreo cookies, small	570	33%	21	12.5	82
Blizzard, Oreo cookies, medium	700	34%	26	16	102
Blizzard, Oreo cookies, large	1010	34%	37	23	146
Buster bar, 1	450	58%	28	13	39
Chocolate dilly bar, 1	210	57%	13	7	21
Classic banana split, 1	510	20%	12	8	93
Curly shake, chocolate, small	620	26%	18	11.5	101
Curly shake, chocolate, large	1200	26%	34	23	195
Curly shake, strawberry, small	540	30%	17	11.5	84
Curly shake, strawberry, large	1040	29%	33	22	163
DQ fudge bar, 1	50	0%	0	0	13
DQ vanilla orange bar, 1	60	0%	0	0	17
Misty, cherry, small	210	0%	0	0	58
Misty, cherry, large	430	0%	0	0	116

Product and Portion Size	Calories	% Cal from Fat	Total Fat (g)	Bad Fat (g)	Net Carbs (g)
Misty, grape, small	240	0%	0	0	66
Misty, grape, large	480	0%	0	0	132
Misty, lemon lime, small	140	0%	0	0	38
Misty, lemon lime, large	280	0%	0	0	76
Peanut butter Blast, 1	700	48%	37	19	77
Pecan Praline Parfait, 1	720	36%	29	11.5	104
Starkiss bar, 1	80	0%	0	0	21
Strawberry shortcake, 1	430	28%	14	10	69
Sundae, chocolate, small	280	21%	7	4.5	40
Sundae, chocolate, large	580	24%	15	10	99
Sundae, strawberry, small	240	25%	7	4.5	40
Sundae, strawberry, large	500	26%	15	9	82
Vanilla cone, small	230	26%	7	4.5	38
Vanilla cone, medium	330	27%	9	6	53
Vanilla cone, large	480	27%	15	9.5	76
Sandwiches, Sides					
Bacon cheeseburger, 1	750	55%	46	23	46
Buffalo chicken strips, 4 strips	540	50%	30	12	33

Product and Portion Size	Calories	% Cal from Fat	Total Fat (g)	Bad Fat (g)	Net Carbs (g)
Buttermilk dressing, reduced calorie, 1 packet	140	86%	13	2	5
California grillburger, 1	690	58%	44	17	43
Chicken quesadilla, 1	550	51%	31	19	32
Chicken strips, no sauce, 4 strips	400	53%	24	9.5	18
Classic grillburger, no cheese, 1	600	48%	33	15	47
Classic hot dog, 1	400	60%	27	12.5	25
Classic hot dog, chili cheese, 1	510	61%	35	17	27
Crispy chicken salad, no dressing or croutons, 1	350	51%	20	8.5	15
Crispy chicken sandwich, 1	520	46%	26	6.5	44
DQ Honey mustard dressing, 1 packet	260	73%	21	3.5	18
Fish fillets, no sauce, 4	440	50%	24	13	40
French fries, 5 oz	380	37%	15	7	52
French fries, 7 oz	530	36%	21	10	72
Grilled chicken salad, 1	240	38%	10	5	8
Grilled chicken sandwich, 1	520	46%	26	6.5	44
Grilled turkey sandwich, 1	730	55%	45	15	44
Half lb. grillburger, no cheese, 1	860	56%	53	26	27
House salad, no dressing or croutons, 1	120	38%	5	3	8

Product and Portion Size	Calories	% Cal from Fat	Total Fat (g)	Bad Fat (g)	Net Carbs (g)
Onion rings, 4 oz	470	57%	30	13	42
Onion rings, 5 oz	590	57%	37	16	52
Vegetable quesadilla, 1	440	50%	25	15	31
FAST FOOD—Dunkin Donuts					
Bagels					
Cinnamon raisin, 1	330	9%	3	0.5	62
Everything, 1	370	14%	6	0.5	64
Multigrain, 1	380	13%	6	1	63
Plain, 1	320	7%	2.5	0.5	60
Sesame, 1	380	18%	8	0.5	61
Wheat, 1	330	11%	4	1	58
Bakery					
Apple Danish, 1	330	55%	20	9	31
Banana walnut muffin, 1	540	43%	25	3.5	66
Biscuit, 1	250	48%	13	11.5	28
Blueberry muffin, 1	470	32%	17	3	71
Cheese Danish, 1	340	59%	22	10	29
Chocolate chip muffin, 1	630	38%	26	8	87

Product and Portion Size	Calories	% Cal from Fat	Total Fat (g)	Bad Fat (g)	Net Carbs (g)
Chocolate chunk cookie, 2 cookies	220	45%	11	7	27
Chocolate chunk cookie w/walnuts, 2 cookies	230	48%	12	6	26
Coffee cake muffin, 1	580	29%	19	3	77
Corn muffin, 1	510	31%	18	3.5	76
Oatmeal raisin pecan cookie, 2 cookies	220	41%	10	5	28
Plain croissant, 1	330	52%	18	11.5	37
Beverages					
Cappuccino, 10 oz	80	50%	4.5	2.5	7
Caramel crème latte, 10 oz	260	31%	9	6	40
Caramel swirl latte, w/soy, 10 oz	210	14%	3.5	9	33
Coffee Coolatta, w/2% milk, 16 oz	190	11%	2	1.5	41
Coffee Coolatta, w/cream, 16 oz	350	54%	22	14	40
Dunkaccino, 10 oz	230	39%	10	8	35
Espresso, 2 oz	0	0%	0	0	1
Flavored coffees, all, 10 oz	20	0%	0	0	4
Hot latte, lite, 10 oz	70	0%	0	0	10
Iced coffee w/cream, 16 oz	70	71%	6	3.5	4
Iced coffee w/skim milk & sugar, 16 oz	70	0%	0	0	16

Product and Portion Size	Calories	% Cal from Fat	Total Fat (g)	Bad Fat (g)	Net Carbs (g)
Iced latte w/skim milk, 16 oz	70	0%	0	0	11
Latte w/soy milk, 10 oz	90	30%	3.5	0	7
Mocha almond iced latte, 16 oz	290	31%	19	7	45
Tropicana Orange Coolatta, 16 oz	370	0%	0	0	89
Turbo hot latte, 10 oz	130	38%	6	3.5	20
Turbo Ice, 16 oz	120	50%	7	3.5	14
Vanilla Bean Coolatta, 16 oz	440	34%	17	16	69
Vanilla chai, 10 oz	230	30%	8	6	40
Cream Cheese					
Chive, 2 oz	170	88%	17	11	2
Garden vegetable, 2 oz	170	76%	15	11	4
Lite, 2 oz	110	73%	9	7	6
Salmon, 2 oz	170	88%	17	11	2
Strawberry, 2 oz	190	79%	17	9	9
Donuts and Fancies					
Apple crumb, 1	230	39%	10	3.5	33
Apple fritter, 1	300	43%	14	5.5	40
Apple & spice, 1	200	35%	8	4	28

Product and Portion Size	Calories	% Cal from Fat	Total Fat (g)	Bad Fat (g)	Net Carbs (g)
Bavarian kreme, 1	210	38%	9	4.5	29
Blueberry cake, 1	290	48%	16	6	34
Boston kreme, 1	240	33%	9	5.5	35
Chocolate frosted cake, 1	360	50%	20	10	39
Chocolate frosted donut, 1	200	40%	9	7	28
Chocolate glazed cake, 1	290	48%	16	7.5	32
Chocolate iced bismark, 1	340	38%	15	5	49
Chocolate kreme filled, 1	270	44%	13	7	34
Cinnamon cake donut, 1	330	55%	20	9	33
Cinnamon cake stick, 1	450	60%	30	12	41
Cinnamon cake munchkins, 4	270	48%	15	7.5	30
Coffee roll, 1	270	48%	14	3	32
Éclair, 1	270	37%	11	3	38
French cruller, 1	150	47%	8	5	16
Glazed cake munchkins, 3	280	43%	13	7	37
Glazed cake stick, 1	420	53%	29	12	50
Glazed chocolate cake stick, 1	470	55%	29	12	47
Glazed donut, 1	180	39%	8	5.5	24

Product and Portion Size	Calories	% Cal from Fat	Total Fat (g)	Bad Fat (g)	Net Carbs (g)
Glazed fritter, 1	260	50%	14	5.5	30
Glazed lemon cake, 1	240	50%	14	6	28
Jelly filled donut, 1	210	33%	8	5.5	31
Jelly filled munchkins, 5	210	38%	9	4.5	26
Jelly filled sticks, 1	530	49%	29	12	60
Lemon filled munchkins, 4	170	41%	8	4	23
Maple frosted donut, 1	210	38%	9	4.5	29
Old fashioned cake donut, 1	300	57%	19	9	27
Plain cake munchkins, 4	270	52%	16	8	26
Plain cake stick, 1	420	62%	29	12	34
Powdered cake donut, 1	330	52%	19	9	35
Powdered cake stick, 1	450	58%	29	12	41
Sugar raised donut, 1	170	41%	8	2	21
Sugar raised munchkins, 7	220	50%	12	3	25
Vanilla crème filled, 1	270	44%	13	6.5	35
Sandwiches					
Bacon cheese bagel, 1	540	30%	18	7	67
Bacon egg cheese croissant, 1	520	58%	33	17	40

Product and Portion Size	Calories	% Cal from Fat	Total Fat (g)	Bad Fat (g)	Net Carbs (g)
Egg cheese bagel, 1	470	30%	15	6	63
Ham cheese bagel, 1	510	27%	16	6	24
Ham egg cheese croissant, 1	520	56%	32	17	40
Ham egg cheese English muffin, 1	310	29%	10	5	20
Meatball panini, 1	480	35%	19	9	53
Sausage egg cheese croissant, 1	690	67%	51	24	40
Steak panini, 1	450	24%	12	5.5	27
Southwestern chicken panini, 1	420	21%	10	5	54
Supreme omelet croissant, 1	590	58%	38	19	41
FAST FOOD—Jack in the Box					
Breakfast					
Bacon, egg, cheese biscuit, 1	430	51%	25	13	33
Breakfast Jack, 1	290	38%	12	4.5	28
Chicken biscuit, 1	450	49%	24	12	40
Extreme sausage sandwich, 1	670	64%	48	18.5	29
Meaty breakfast burrito, 1	480	54%	29	11	27
Sausage biscuit, 1	440	59%	29	13	30
Sausage, egg, cheese biscuit, 1	740	66%	55	23	33

Product and Portion Size	Calories	% Cal from Fat	Total Fat (g)	Bad Fat (g)	Net Carbs (g)
Sourdough breakfast sandwich, 1	420	52%	24	10	29
Ultimate breakfast sandwich, 1	570	42%	27	11	47
Salads & Sides					
Asian chicken salad, 1	140	7%	1	0	14
Bacon cheddar potato wedges, 1 serv.	720	60%	48	27	48
Beef monster taco, 1	240	54%	14	7	17
Chicken club salad, 1	300	47%	15	6	9
Natural cut fries, small	270	41%	12	6.5	32
Natural cut fries, large	530	42%	25	13	64
Onion rings, 8	500	54%	30	16	48
Seasoned curly fries, small	270	52%	15	8	27
Seasoned curly fries, large	550	51%	31	16	54
Stuffed jalapenos, 7	530	51%	30	17.5	47
Sandwiches, Entrees					
Bacon bacon cheeseburger, 1	840	60%	56	20.5	49
Bacon chicken sandwich, 1	440	48%	24	8.5	37
Bacon ultimate cheeseburger, 1	1090	64%	77	33	51
Chicken breast strips, 4	500	44%	25	12	33

Product and Portion Size	Calories	% Cal from Fat	Total Fat (g)	Bad Fat (g)	Net Carbs (g)
Fish n chips, small	570	47%	30	16	54
Fish n chips, large	830	46%	42	22	86
Hamburger, 1	310	42%	14	7	29
Hamburger w/cheese, 1	350	46%	17	9	30
Jumbo Jack, 1	600	52%	35	13.5	48
Jumbo Jack w/cheese, 1	690	54%	42	17.5	51
Original Ciabatta burger, 1	710	51%	40	13.5	60
Sourdough grilled chicken club, 1	530	47%	28	9	31
Sourdough Jack, 1	710	65%	51	21	33
Desserts, Shakes					
Cheesecake, 1 serv.	310	45%	16	10	34
Chocolate ice cream shake, 16 oz	880	45%	45	33	106
Oreo cookie ice cream shake, 16 oz	910	48%	49	34	101
Strawberry ice cream shake, 16 oz	880	45%	44	33	105
Vanilla ice cream shake, 16 oz	790	51%	44	33	83
FAST FOOD—KFC					
Sandwiches, Entrees					
Chicken pot pie, 1	770	47%	40	29	65

Product and Portion Size	Calories	% Cal from Fat	Total Fat (g)	Bad Fat (g)	Net Carbs (g)
Crispy strips, 3	400	55%	24	9.5	17
Crispy twists sandwich, 1	670	51%	38	11	52
Double crunch sandwich, 1	530	48%	28	9	39
KFC Snacker, 1	320	47%	16	4.5	29
KFC Snacker sandwich, buffalo, 1	260	27%	8	3.5	30
KFC Snacker sandwich, fish, 1	269	33%	19	3	32
KFC Snacker, ultimate cheese, 1	280	36%	11	4.5	31
Oven roasted chicken, breast, 1	380	45%	19	8.5	11
Oven roasted chicken, drumstick 1	140	50%	8	3	4
Oven roasted chicken, thigh, 1	360	64%	25	8.5	12
Oven roasted chicken, whole wing, 1	150	53%	9	3.5	5
Popcorn chicken, individual	380	50%	1	9.5	23
Popcorn chicken, kids size	270	52%	16	7	15
Popcorn chicken, large	560	50%	31	14	33
Sides, Desserts					
Apple pie minis, 3	400	50%	22	12	21
Apple pie slice	290	34%	11	5.5	42
Baked beans, 1 serv.	230	4%	1	1	15

Product and Portion Size	Calories	% Cal from Fat	Total Fat (g)	Bad Fat (g)	Net Carbs (g)
Baked Cheetos, 1 serv.	120	33%	4.5	1	17
Biscuit, 1	190	47%	10	5.5	23
Fiery buffalo wings, 6	440	52%	26	10.5	23
HBBQ wings, 6	540	56%	33	11.5	35
Hot wings, 6	450	58%	29	10	22
Lil Bucket chocolate cream, 1	270	44%	13	8.5	35
Lil Bucket fudge brownie, 1	270	30%	9	4.5	43
Lil Bucket lemon crème, 1	400	33%	14	8.5	63
Lil Bucket strawberry shortcake, 1	200	25%	6	4	34
Mashed potatoes w/gravy, 1 serv.	130	31%	4.5	1.5	18
Potato wedges, 1 serv.	240	46%	12	7	27
Seasoned rice, 1 serv.	150	7%	1	0	5
Sweet n' spicy wings, 6	460	50%	26	10.5	29
Sweet potato pie, slice	340	41%	16	7	43
FAST FOOD—McDonald's					
Beverages & Desserts					
Apple Dippers w/dip, 1 serv.	100	0%	0.5	0	24
Chocolate triple thick shake, 16 oz	580	16%	10	6.5	75

Product and Portion Size	Calories	% Cal from Fat	Total Fat (g)	Bad Fat (g)	Net Carbs (g)
Deluxe warm cinnamon bun, 1	590	37%	24	13	82
Fruit yogurt parfait, 1	160	11%	2	1	30
McDonaldland cookies, 2 oz	250	29%	8	4.5	41
McFlurry w/M&Ms, 1	620	29%	20	13	95
Orange juice, small	140	0%	0	0	33
Vanilla triple thick shake, 16 oz	550	21%	13	9	96
Breakfast					
Big Breakfast, 1	730	57%	46	21	50
Biscuit, 1	240	41%	11	4.5	30
Egg McMuffin, 1	300	36%	12	4.5	28
Hash browns, 1 serv.	140	51%	8	3.5	13
Hotcakes, margarine & syrup, 1 serv.	600	26%	17	8	100
Sausage burritto, 1	300	48%	16	7	25
Sausage, egg, cheese McGriddle, 1 serv.	560	51%	32	12.5	46
Sausage McMuffin, 1	380	52%	22	8.5	29
Sausage McMuffin w/egg, 1	450	54%	27	10.5	29
Sausage patty, 1	170	79%	15	6	2
Scrambled Eggs (2)	190	57%	12	4	5

Product and Portion Size	Calories	% Cal from Fat	Total Fat (g)	Bad Fat (g)	Net Carbs (g)
Sandwiches, Sides					
Bacon ranch salad grilled chicken, 1	260	31%	9	4	9
Big Mac, 1	560	48%	30	11.5	44
Big N Tasty, 1	470	44%	23	9.5	38
Caesar salad w/crispy chicken, 1	300	39%	13	5.5	19
California Cobb salad w/grilled chicken, 1	280	35%	11	5	8
Cheeseburger, 1	310	35%	12	7	34
Chicken Selects breast strips, 3 pcs	380	47%	20	6	28
Chicken McNuggets, 6 pcs	250	54%	15	4.5	15
Double cheeseburger, 1	460	45%	23	12.5	36
Fillet-O-Fish, 1	400	41%	18	5	41
French fries, small	250	47%	13	6	27
French fries, medium	380	47%	20	9	42
French fries, large	570	47%	30	14	63
Fruit & walnut salad, 1	310	38%	13	2	38
McChicken, 1	370	39%	16	4.5	40
Premium grilled chicken classic sandwich, 1	420	19%	9	2	49
Premium grilled chicken club sandwich, 1	590	34%	22	8	61

Product and Portion Size	Calories	% Cal from Fat	Total Fat (g)	Bad Fat (g)	Net Carbs (g)
Quarterpounder w/o cheese, 1	420	39%	18	8	37
Quarterpounder w/cheese, 1	510	44%	25	13.5	40
FAST FOOD—Panda Express					
BBQ Pork, 5.5 oz	400	52%	23	9	14
Beef w/broccoli, 5.5 oz	150	40%	7	1.5	7
Chicken egg roll, 1	170	42%	8	1.5	6
Chicken w/mushrooms, 5.5 oz	130	42%	6	1.5	8
Chicken w/string beans, 5.5 oz	160	45%	8	1.5	8
Egg flower soup, 12 oz	88	25%	2.2	0	16
Firecracker beef, 5.5 oz	160	45%	8	2	7
Fried shrimp, 6 pcs	260	45%	13	2.5	25
Hot and sour soup, 12 oz	110	29%	3.5	1	12
Kung Pao Chicken, 5.5 oz	240	54%	15	3	11
Kung Pao Shrimp, 5.5 oz	260	45%	13	2.5	25
Mandarin chicken, 5.5 oz	250	36%	10	3	8
Mandarin sauce, 1.5 oz	70	0%	0	0	17
Mixed vegetables, 5.5 oz	50	27%	1.5	0	4
Orange flavored chicken, 5.5 oz	500	49%	27	6.5	39

Product and Portion Size	Calories	% Cal from Fat	Total Fat (g)	Bad Fat (g)	Net Carbs (g)
Steamed rice, 8 oz	380	6%	2.5	0.5	78
Sweet & sour pork, 5.5 oz	400	52%	23	4.5	33
Sweet & sour sauce, 1.5 oz	80	0%	0	0	17
Tangy shrimp w/pineapple, 5.5 oz	150	30%	5	1	7
Vegetable chow mein, 8 oz	390	28%	12	2	52
Vegetable fried rice, 8 oz	450	28%	14	3	61
Veggie spring roll, 1	80	39%	3.5	1	9
FAST FOOD—Starbucks					
Desserts/Baked Goods					
Apple fritter, 1	790	43%	37	19	98
Banana nut loaf, 1 pc	360	44%	18	11	46
Banana walnut muffin, 1	460	43%	22	5	59
Black bottom cupcake, 1	580	47%	29	9	70
Black & white cookie, 1	430	35%	17	4	66
Blueberry muffin, 1	420	43%	20	5	54
Blueberry scone, 1	500	52%	29	18	55
Bran muffin, 1	420	40%	19	2	52
Butter croissant, 1	440	52%	25	16	43

Product and Portion Size	Calories	% Cal from Fat	Total Fat (g)	Bad Fat (g)	Net Carbs (g)
Chocolate marshmallow bar, 1	510	47%	27	14	59
Cinnamon nut croissant, 1	320	69%	24	12	21
Cinnamon twist, 1	320	47%	17	2.5	36
Cranberry muffin, 1	460	46%	23	5	45
Cream cheese Danish, 1	440	70%	34	17	59
Crumb cake, 1	430	53%	25	24	45
Fudge brownie, 1	380	37%	15	6	56
Iced lemon pound cake, 1	500	40%	23	12	68
Maple nut scone, 1	650	48%	34	19	77
Multigrain bagel, 1	360	10%	4	0	68
Orange cupcake, 1	310	42%	15	6.5	41
Sesame bagel, 1	280	0%	0	0	56
Seven layer bar, 1	600	55%	37	19.5	59
Starbucks expresso brownie, 1	370	51%	21	13	41
Tomato & asiago focaccia, 1	410	39%	18	5	45
Beverages					
Banana caramel Frappuccino, no whip, 16 oz	410	9%	3.5	2.5	89
Caffe latte, 16 oz	260	46%	14	9	21

Product and Portion Size	Calories	% Cal from Fat	Total Fat (g)	Bad Fat (g)	Net Carbs (g)
Caffe vanilla Frappuccino, no whip, 16 oz	340	9%	3.5	2	72
Cappuccino, 16 oz	150	47%	8	5	13
Caramel apple cider, no whip, 16 oz	300	0%	0	0	72
Iced caffe latte, 16 oz	160	44%	8	5	13
Iced caffe mocha, whip, 16 oz	350	51%	20	12.5	35
Iced Tazo green tea latte, 16 oz	250	28%	8	4.5	36
Tazo black tea lemonade, 16 oz	120	0%	0	0	30
Tazo chai tea latte, 16 oz	290	21%	7	4.5	50
Toffee nut crème w/whip, 16 oz	450	49%	24	15	43
Vanilla latte, 16 oz	320	34%	12	7	39
FAST FOOD—Subway					
6-inch Sandwiches					
Cheese steak, 1	360	25%	10	4.5	42
Chicken & bacon ranch, 1	530	43%	25	10.5	42
Chicken parmesan, 1	510	33%	18	6	59
Cold cut combo, 1	410	37%	17	7.5	43
Ham, 1	290	16%	5	1.5	43
Italian BMT, 1	450	42%	21	8	43

Product and Portion Size	Calories	% Cal from Fat	Total Fat (g)	Bad Fat (g)	Net Carbs (g)
Meatball marinara, 1	560	39%	24	12	56
Oven roasted chicken breast, 1	330	15%	5	1.5	43
Roast beef, 1	290	16%	5	2	41
Spicy Italian, 1	480	48%	25	9	42
Tuna, 1	530	53%	31	7.5	43
Turkey breast, 1	280	14%	4.5	1.5	42
Turkey breast & ham, 1	290	16%	5	1.5	43
Veggie Delite, 1	230	13%	3	1	40
6-Inch Double Meat					
Cheese steak, 1	450	27%	14	6	44
Chipotle Southwest cheese steak, 1	540	39%	24	7	44
Classic tuna, 1	790	62%	55	12	41
Cold cut combo, 1	550	45%	28	11	45
Ham, 1	380	18%	7	2.5	53
Italian BMT, 1	630	49%	35	14	45
Meatball marinara, 1	960	40%	42	20	72
Oven roasted chicken, 1	430	16%	8	3	46
Seafood sensation, 1	640	35%	38	9	53

Product and Portion Size	Calories	% Cal from Fat	Total Fat (g)	Bad Fat (g)	Net Carbs (g)
Subway club, 1	420	19%	8	3.5	44
Turkey breast, 1	340	15%	6	1.5	44
Turkey breast & ham, 1	360	17%	7	3	46
Turkey breast, ham & bacon melt, 1	500	30%	17	8	47
Breakfast Sandwiches & Wraps					
Cheese sandwich, 1	310	26%	9	3.5	40
Cheese wrap, 1	220	41%	10	3.5	8
Chipotle steak & cheese sandwich, 1	510	45%	25	9	42
Chipotle steak & cheese wrap, 1	430	56%	10	3.5	8
Double bacon & cheese sandwich, 1	500	42%	23	12.5	41
Double bacon & cheese wrap, 1	420	55%	25	11.5	10
Honey mustard ham & egg sandwich, 1	310	16%	5	1.5	47
Honey mustard ham & egg wrap, 1	230	26%	7	1	15
Western with cheese sandwich, 1	400	33%	14	7	42
Western with cheese wrap, 1	310	45%	16	6	11
Deli-style Sandwiches					
Ham, 1	210	17%	4	1.5	33
Roast beef, 1	220	18%	4.5	2	32

Product and Portion Size	Calories	% Cal from Fat	Total Fat (g)	Bad Fat (g)	Net Carbs (g)
Turkey breast, 1	210	17%	3.5	1.5	33
Tuna w/cheese, 1	350	49%	18	5.5	32
Desserts & Beverages					
Apple pie, 1	245	39%	10	2	36
Berry Lishus, small	110	0%	0	0	27
Berry Lishus w/banana, small	140	0%	0	0	33
Chocolate chip cookie, 1	210	43%	10	5	29
Chocolate chunk cookie, 1	220	41%	10	6	29
Double chocolate chip cookie, 1	210	43%	10	5	29
Fruit roll up, 1	50	10%	1	0	12
M&M cookie, 1	210	43%	10	6	29
Oatmeal raisin cookie, 1	200	35%	8	5	28
Peanut butter cookie, 1	220	50%	12	5	25
Pineapple delight beverage, small	130	0%	0	0	33
Pineapple delight w/banana, small	160	0%	0	0	38
Sugar cookie, 1	230	48%	12	7	28
Sunrise Refresher beverage, small	120	0%	0	0	28
White chip macadamia nut cookie, 1	245	39%	10	2	36

Product and Portion Size	Calories	% Cal from Fat	Total Fat (g)	Bad Fat (g)	Net Carbs (g)
Soups					
Brown & wild rice w/chicken, 10 oz	230	48%	11	3.5	25
Chicken & dumpling, 10 oz	140	25%	3.5	1.5	18
Cream of broccoli, 10 oz	140	36%	5	2	14
Cream of potato w/bacon, 10 oz	220	45%	10	4	23
Golden broccoli & cheese, 10 oz	180	56%	11	5	12
Minestrone, 10 oz	90	9%	1	0	14
New England style clam chowder, 10 oz	150	33%	5	1.5	18
Roasted chicken noodle, 10 oz	90	28%	2	0.5	11
Spanish style chicken w/rice, 10 oz	110	25%	2.5	1	15
Tomato garden vegetable w/rotini, 10 oz	90	6%	0.5	0	17
Vegetable beef, 10 oz	100	20%	1.5	0.5	14
Wraps					
Chicken & bacon ranch w/cheese, 1	440	44%	27	10.5	9
Turkey breast, 1	190	26%	6	1	9
Turkey breast & bacon melt, 1	380	58%	24	7	11
Tuna w/cheese, 1	440	66%	32	6.5	7

FAST FOOD—Taco Bell

Product and Portion Size	Calories	% Cal from Fat	Total Fat (g)	Bad Fat (g)	Net Carbs (g)
Burritos					
Bean burrito, 1	370	24%	10	5.5	47
Burrito supreme, beef, 1	440	37%	18	10	47
Burrito supreme, chicken, 1	410	31%	14	8	45
Burrito supreme, steak, 1	420	34%	16	9	44
Chili cheese burrito, 1	390	42%	18	10.5	37
Grilled stuft burrito, beef, 1	720	40%	32	14	73
Grilled stuft burrito, chicken, 1	670	34%	25	9.5	70
Grilled stuft burrito, steak, 1	680	36%	27	11	70
One-half lb beef combo burrito, 1	470	36%	19	9	47
One-half lb beef & potato burrito, 1	540	42%	25	11.5	62
One-half lb cheesy bean & rice burrito, 1	490	39%	21	9	55
Seven-layer buritto, 1	530	36%	21	10.5	59
Spicy chicken burrito, 1	420	41%	19	5.5	47
Chalupas					
Nacho cheese, beef, 1	380	52%	22	8	31
Nacho cheese, chicken, 1	350	46%	18	7	29
Nacho cheese, steak, 1	360	50%	20	7.5	29

Product and Portion Size	Calories	% Cal from Fat	Total Fat (g)	Bad Fat (g)	Net Carbs (g)
Supreme, beef, 1	400	54%	24	10.5	29
Supreme, chicken, 1	370	51%	21	9	27
Supreme, steak, 1	370	54%	22	9	27
Gorditas					
Baja, beef, fresco, 1	250	32%	9	3	28
Baja, chicken, regular, 1	320	42%	15	3.5	27
Baja, steak, regular, 1	320	45%	16	4	27
Supreme, beef, fresco, 1	250	32%	9	3	28
Supreme, beef, regular, 1	350	49%	19	5.5	29
Supreme, chicken, fresco, 1	230	23%	6	1	26
Supreme, chicken, regular, 1	290	37%	12	5	26
Supreme, steak, fresco, 1	230	27%	7	1.5	26
Supreme, steak, regular, 1	290	40%	13	6.5	26
Tacos					
Chicken ranchero taco, fresco, 1	170	21%	4	1.5	18
Chicken ranchero taco, regular, 1	270	47%	14	4.5	19
Double decker taco, 1	340	37%	14	6.5	34
Grande soft taco, 1	450	42%	21	10.5	42

Product and Portion Size	Calories	% Cal from Fat	Total Fat (g)	Bad Fat (g)	Net Carbs (g)
Grilled steak soft taco, fresco, 1	170	26%	5	2	19
Grilled steak soft taco, regular, 1	280	55%	17	5.5	20
Soft taco, beef, fresco, 1	190	38%	8	3	20
Soft taco, beef, regular, 1	210	43%	10	5	19
Taco, fresco style, 1	150	42%	7	3	12
Taco, regular style, 1	170	53%	10	4.5	12
Miscellaneous					
Cheese quesadilla, 1	490	51%	28	15	36
Cheesy fiesta potatoes, 1 serv.	290	56%	18	9	26
Chicken quesadilla, 1	540	50%	30	15	37
Cinnamon twists, 1	160	28%	5	2	26
Crunchwrap supreme, 1	560	39%	24	12.5	66
Enchirito, beef, 1	380	43%	18	10.5	30
Enchirito, chicken, 1	350	36%	14	8.5	28
Enchirito, steak, 1	360	40%	16	9.5	28
Express taco salad, 1	630	49%	34	15.5	48
Fiesta taco salad, 1	860	48%	46	19	70
Fiesta taco salad, no shell, 1	490	46%	25	13	33

Product and Portion Size	Calories	% Cal from Fat	Total Fat (g)	Bad Fat (g)	Net Carbs (g)
Mexican pizza, 1	540	52%	31	13.5	42
Mexican rice, 1 serv.	200	41%	9	4	24
Nachos, BellGrande, 1	790	50%	44	19	69
Nachos, supreme, 1	460	51%	26	11.5	37
SW steak border bowl, 1	690	37%	28	10.5	69
Tostada, 1	250	36%	10	5.5	22
Zesty chicken border bowl, 1	730	49%	40	10.5	59
FAST FOOD—Wendy's					
Biggie French fries, 5.6 oz	490	43%	24	10	58
Blackforest ham & swiss frescata, 1	480	38%	20	6	46
Cheeseburger, jr	320	34%	13	6.5	33
Chicken BLT, 1	340	47%	18	9	8
Chili, large	330	24%	9	4	27
Fix 'n mix frosty, medium	170	21%	4	2.5	29
Frosty, medium	430	23%	11	7	74
Ham & cheese sandwich, kids	240	25%	6	3	31
Hamburger, jr.	280	29%	9	5	33
Homestyle chicken fillet sandwich	540	35%	22	5.5	55

Product and Portion Size	Calories	% Cal from Fat	Total Fat (g)	Bad Fat (g)	Net Carbs (g)
Homestyle chicken strips, 3 strips	410	39%	18	6.5	33
Low-fat strawberry flavored yogurt, 1	140	7%	1.5	1	27
Mandarin chicken salad, 1	170	9%	2	0.5	15
Nuggets, 10 pcs	440	59%	29	9.5	25
Roasted turkey & basil pesto frescata, 1	420	33%	16	3	46
Side salad, 1	35	0%	0	0	6
Southwest taco salad, 1	440	45%	22	13	23
Spicy chicken fillet sandwich, 1	510	33%	19	5	55
Ultimate chicken grill sandwich, 1	360	17%	7	1.5	42
FIGS					
Canned, 1 cup solids & liquid	131	2%	0	0	30
Fresh, large 2.5"	47	3%	0	0	10
Stewed, 1 cup	277	3%	1	0	60
Sun-Maid, mission & calimyrna, 4 figs	120	0%	0	0	23
FILBERTS, dry roasted, no salt, 1 oz	**182**	**81%**	**18**	**1**	**2**
FLOUNDER, baked, 3 oz	99	12%	1	0	0
Mrs. Paul's fillets, 1 fillet	150	47%	7	3.5	12

Product and Portion Size	Calories	% Cal from Fat	Total Fat (g)	Bad Fat (g)	Net Carbs (g)
FLOUR					
Barley, 1 cup	511	4%	2	0	95
Corn, whole grain, yellow, 1 cup	422	9%	5	1	74
Cornmeal, self-rising, enriched, 1 cup	592	7%	5	1	114
Gold Medal Better for Bread, ¼ cup	100	0%	0	0	21
Gold Medal unbleached, all-purpose, ¼ cup	100	0%	0	0	21
Gold Medal whole wheat, ¼ cup	100	5%	0.5	0.5	18
Rice, brown, 1 cup	574	6%	4	1	114
Rye, dark, 1 cup	415	7%	3	0	59
FRANKFURTERS					
Ballpark					
Beef franks, 1	180	83%	16	7	3
Bun size smoked white turkey, 1	45	0%	0	0	5
Fat free franks, 1	40	0%	0	0	4
Grillmaster deli style 1	250	80%	23	9	3
Grillmaster hearty beef, 1	250	80%	23	9	3
Lite beef, 1	100	70%	7	3	3

Product and Portion Size	Calories	% Cal from Fat	Total Fat (g)	Bad Fat (g)	Net Carbs (g)
Hebrew National					
97% f-f beef, 1	45	30%	1.5	1	3
¼-lb dinner frank, 1	350	83%	32	15	5
Beef frank, 1	150	87%	14	6	1
Cocktail franks, 5 links	180	83%	16	7	1
Frank in a blanket, 5 links	290	76%	24	10	7
Oscar Mayer					
Beef bun-length, 1	180	83%	17	8	2
Beef franks, 1	140	86%	13	7	1
Beef jumbo, 1	180	83%	17	8	2
Beef light, 1	90	67%	6	6	2
Beef XXL deli style, 1	230	87%	22	10.5	1
Cheese dogs, 1	140	86%	13	4	1
Turkey franks, 1	100	70%	8	2.5	2
Wieners, f-f, 1	40	0%	0	0	3
Wieners, jumbo, 1	170	82%	16	5	0
XXL hot & spicy, 1	210	81%	19	8	1

Product and Portion Size	Calories	% Cal from Fat	Total Fat (g)	Bad Fat (g)	Net Carbs (g)
FRANKFURTER SUBSTITUTES					
Morningstar corn dog, 1	150	20%	4	0.5	21
Morningstar veggie dog, 1	80	6%	0.5	0	5
Worthington corn dog, 1	150	20%	4	0.5	19
Worthington little links, 2 links	90	50%	5	0.5	1
Worthington low-fat big franks, 1	80	25%	2.5	0.5	1
Yves, hot & spicy chili veggie, 1	74	12%	1	0	3
Yves, tofu dog, 1	47	10%	0.5	0	2
Yves, veggie dog, 1	56	0%	0	0	1
FRENCH TOAST					
Aunt Jemima cinnamon French toast, 2 slices	240	21%	6	1.5	37
Murry's French toast sticks, 5 sticks	300	33%	11	2	47
Pillsbury French toast sticks, cinnamon, 6 sticks	350	17%	6	3.5	68
Pillsbury French toast sticks, homestyle, 6 sticks	310	19%	6	3.5	67
FROSTING					
Betty Crocker					
Homestyle fluffy white, f-f, 6 Tbs prep.	100	0%	0	0	24
Rich & Creamy butter cream, 2 Tbs	150	47%	7	4.5	20

Product and Portion Size	Calories	% Cal from Fat	Total Fat (g)	Bad Fat (g)	Net Carbs (g)
Rich & Creamy caramel, 2 Tbs	150	47%	7	4.5	20
Rich & Creamy cherry, 2 Tbs	150	47%	7	4.5	21
Rich & Creamy chocolate, 2 Tbs	140	50%	7	4.5	17
Rich & Creamy coconut pecan, 2 Tbs	140	50%	7	4.5	17
Rich & Creamy cream cheese, 2 Tbs	150	47%	7	4.5	20
Rich & Creamy lemon, 2 Tbs	150	47%	8	5.5	20
Rich & Creamy rainbow chip, 2 Tbs	140	32%	5	3.5	23
Rich & Creamy triple choc. fudge chip, 2 Tbs	140	32%	5	3	23
Rich & Creamy vanilla, 2 Tbs	150	47%	7	4.5	21
Whipped butter cream, 2 Tbs	110	41%	5	3	15
Whipped chocolate, 2 Tbs	100	45%	5	2.5	14
Whipped chocolate mousse, 2 Tbs	90	44%	4.5	2.5	13
Whipped cream cheese, 2 Tbs	110	41%	5	3	15
Whipped lemon, 2 Tbs	110	41%	5	3	15
Whipped milk chocolate, 2 Tbs	100	40%	4.5	2.5	14
Whipped vanilla, 2 Tbs	110	41%	5	3	15
Whipped whipped cream, 2 Tbs	100	45%	5	3	15

Product and Portion Size	Calories	% Cal from Fat	Total Fat (g)	Bad Fat (g)	Net Carbs (g)
FROZEN BREAKFAST (also see “French Toast” and “Pancakes”)					
Amy’s Kitchen, breakfast burrito, 1	250	28%	7	0.5	33
Jimmy Dean Omelet, 3 cheese, 1	270	70%	21	10	4
Jimmy Dean Omelet, ham & cheese, 1	280	54%	17	7	5
Jimmy Dean Omelet, sausage & cheese, 1	270	74%	22	8	4
Jimmy Dean Omelet, western style, 1	270	48%	14	4.5	4
Jimmy Dean wrap, sausage, egg, cheese, 1	320	50%	17	7.5	24
Morningstar Farms breakfast sand. w/cheese, 1	250	10%	3	0.5	30
Pillsbury Toaster Scrambles, bacon & sausage, 1	180	56%	12	4.5	15
Pillsbury Toaster Scrambles, cheese, egg, bacon, 1	180	56%	12	4.5	15
Pillsbury Toaster Scrambles, cheese, egg, sausage 1	180	56%	11	4.5	15
South Beach Diet breakfast wrap, all-American, 1	200	40%	9	4	11
South Beach Diet breakfast wrap, Denver, 1	180	30%	7	3	12
South Beach Diet breakfast wrap, SW style, 1	160	31%	5	2.5	11
South Beach Diet breakfast wrap, vegetable, 1	160	31%	3	0.5	30
FROZEN DINNERS & ENTREES					
Amy’s Kitchen					
Asian noodle stir-fry, 1 pkg	290	21%	7	1	40

Product and Portion Size	Calories	% Cal from Fat	Total Fat (g)	Bad Fat (g)	Net Carbs (g)
Black bean veg. enchilada, 1	180	28%	6	0.5	44
Broccoli pot pie, 1	430	44%	22	10	42
Brown rice, black-eyed peas, veg. bowl, 1	290	35%	11	1.5	30
Brown rice & vegetables bowl, 1	260	30%	9	1	31
Country vegetable pie, 1	370	38%	16	9	43
Indian Mattar paneer, 1 pkg	320	22%	8	1.5	49
Indian samosa wraps, 1 wrap	260	27%	8	1	34
Indian vegetable korma, 1 pkg	300	33%	12	3.5	34
Macaroni & cheese, 1 pkg	410	34%	16	10	44
Mexican casserole bowl, 1	470	30%	16	5	63
Mexican tamale pie, 1	150	20%	3	0	23
Nondairy vegetable pot pie, 1	360	33%	13	1.5	45
Pesto tortelli bowl, 1	430	40%	19	8	42
Ravioli bowl, 1	380	26%	12	4.5	51
Rice macaroni & cheese, 1 pkg	400	35%	16	10	44
Santa Fe enchilada bowl, 1	350	29%	11	2	37
Shepherd's pie, 1	160	22%	4	0	22
Stuffed pasta shells bowl, 1	310	39%	13	7	25

Product and Portion Size	Calories	% Cal from Fat	Total Fat (g)	Bad Fat (g)	Net Carbs (g)
Teriyaki bowl, 1	290	14%	4.5	0.5	48
Thai noodle stir-fry, 1 pkg	310	32%	11	7	40
Tofu vegetable lasagna, 1 pkg	300	30%	10	1.5	35
Vegetable pot pie, 1	420	40%	19	12	50
Whole Meals: Black bean enchilada, 1 meal	330	21%	8	1	44
Whole Meals: Cheese enchilada, 1 meal	350	40%	15	7	32
Whole Meals: chili & cornbread, 1 meal	340	18%	6	2.5	49
Whole Meals: Country dinner, 1 meal	390	28%	12	4	52
Whole Meals: Veggie loaf, 1 meal	280	21%	7	1	40
Bertolli					
Grilled chicken alfredo, ½ pkg	710	54%	42	23.5	50
Roast chicken & linguini, ½ pkg	420	36%	17	4.5	37
Shrimp, asparagus & penne, ½ pkg	480	40%	21	9	46
Birds Eye—Voila!					
Alfredo chicken, 1 cup cooked	320	47%	17	10	24
Beef steak & garlic potatoes, 1 cup cooked	190	32%	7	2	17
Chicken fajita, 1 cup cooked	150	33%	6	2	10
Chicken & sausage, reduced carbs, 1 cup cooked	170	41%	8	2.5	6

Product and Portion Size	Calories	% Cal from Fat	Total Fat (g)	Bad Fat (g)	Net Carbs (g)
Chicken stir-fry, 1 cup cooked	160	16%	3	1.5	20
Garden herb chicken, 1 cup cooked	280	36%	11	6	27
Garlic chicken, 1 cup cooked	240	29%	8	3	18
Garlic shrimp, 1 cup cooked	220	36%	8	3.5	25
Pesto chicken primavera, 1 cup cooked	210	29%	7	3	22
Teriyaki beef & veg., reduced carb, 1 cup cooked	160	22%	4	1.5	11
Teriyaki chicken, 1 cup cooked	250	10%	2.5	0	42
Three cheese chicken, 1 cup cooked	210	33%	8	3.5	19
Gorton's					
Alfredo fillet meal, 1	160	16%	3	1.5	9
Alfredo shrimp bowl, 1	250	18%	5	1.5	35
Beer batter fillets, 2 fillets	230	57%	14	2.5	18
Classic grilled salmon, 1 fillet	100	30%	3.5	0.5	15
Crispy battered fillets, 2 fillets	260	58%	17	3	17
Crunchy golden fillets, 2 fillets	240	46%	12	2.5	23
Fish sticks, 6	250	52%	14	3.5	11
Fried rice shrimp bowl, 1	350	7%	2.5	0.5	67
Garlic & herb fish fillets, 2 fillets	230	48%	12	2	22

Product and Portion Size	Calories	% Cal from Fat	Total Fat (g)	Bad Fat (g)	Net Carbs (g)
Grilled fillets, Caesar parmesan, 1 fillet	100	25%	3	0.5	1
Grilled fillets, Cajun blackened, 1 fillet	100	25%	3	0.5	1
Grilled fillets, lemon pepper, 1 fillet	100	25%	3	0.5	1
Lemon & herb butter fillet, 1 meal	240	13%	3.5	1	31
Original batter tenders, 4 oz	270	52%	15	3	25
Parmesan breaded fillets, 2 fillets	250	56%	15	3	19
Popcorn fish, 11 pcs	280	54%	17	4.5	22
Popcorn shrimp, beer batter, 18 shrimp	270	52%	16	4.5	24
Popcorn shrimp, original, 20 shrimp	240	46%	12	3.5	24
Primavera shrimp bowl, 1	270	19%	6	2.5	40
Ranch fillets, 2 fillets	240	50%	13	2.5	22
Teriyaki shrimp bowl, 1	320	16%	6	1	55
Green Giant—Complete Skillet Meals					
Chicken alfredo, 1¼ cup prep.	270	15%	4.5	3	34
Chicken & cheesy pasta, 1¼ cup prep.	270	19%	6	3	34
Chicken lo mein, 1 cup prep.	190	9%	2	0	28
Chicken teriyaki, 1½ cup prep.	240	4%	1	0	43
Garlic chicken pasta, 1 cup prep.	230	23%	6	2.5	29

Product and Portion Size	Calories	% Cal from Fat	Total Fat (g)	Bad Fat (g)	Net Carbs (g)
Sweet & sour chicken, 1¼ cup prep.	320	5%	1.5	0	59
Green Giant Create-A-Meal					
Spicy Teriyaki, 1 cup prep.	210	29%	7	1	13
Stir-Fry lo mein, 1 cup prep.	270	26%	7	1.5	26
Stir-Fry sesame, 1 cup prep.	260	42%	12	2	8
Sweet 'n Sour, 1 cup prep.	280	21%	7	1	33
Szechuan, 1 cup prep.	190	42%	9	2.5	7
Teriyaki, 1 cup prep.	180	33%	6	1	8
Healthy Choice, Complete Selections					
Asiago chicken portobello, 1 pkg	330	18%	6	2.5	41
Beef pot roast, 1 pkg	310	23%	7	3	40
Beef stroganoff, 1 pkg	340	26%	9	2	39
Charbroiled beef patty, 1 pkg	310	26%	9	3	31
Chicken broccoli alfredo, 1 pkg	300	15%	5	2	38
Chicken enchilada, 1 pkg	310	19%	7	2.5	40
Chicken parmegiana, 1 pkg	320	28%	9	3	34
Chicken teriyaki, 1 pkg	280	14%	4	1	38
Country breaded chicken, 1 pkg	370	24%	9	2	47

Product and Portion Size	Calories	% Cal from Fat	Total Fat (g)	Bad Fat (g)	Net Carbs (g)
Creamy garlic shrimp, 1 pkg	280	18%	5	1.5	39
Grilled turkey breast, 1 pkg	250	18%	5	2	26
Herb baked fish, 1 pkg	360	19%	8	2	50
Honey glazed chicken, 1 pkg	270	22%	6	2	26
Lemon pepper fish, 1 pkg	280	16%	5	2	42
Oven roasted beef, 1 pkg	280	25%	7	2.5	28
Roasted chicken breast, 1 pkg	290	24%	7	2	29
Sesame chicken, 1 pkg	330	21%	8	2	33
Stuffed pasta shells, 1 pkg	290	21%	6	3	33
Sweet & sour chicken, 1 pkg	350	26%	9	3	44
Traditional turkey breast, 1 pkg	300	13%	4	1	36
Healthy Choice, Simple Selections					
Beef teriyaki, 1 pkg	310	23%	7	2.5	39
Cheesy rice & chicken, 1 pkg	220	27%	6	2.5	19
Chicken breast & vegetables, 1 pkg	270	30%	7	2	24
Chicken fettuccini alfredo, 1 pkg	210	24%	5	2	18
Chicken piccata, 1 pkg	270	17%	5	2.5	37
Chicken rigatoni, 1 pkg	250	28%	7	2	25

Product and Portion Size	Calories	% Cal from Fat	Total Fat (g)	Bad Fat (g)	Net Carbs (g)
Grilled chicken & mashed potatoes, 1 pkg	160	22%	3.5	1.5	15
Lasagna bake, 1 pkg	270	26%	7	2.5	34
Macaroni & cheese, 1 pkg	210	19%	4	2	28
Manicotti w/4 cheeses, 1 pkg	270	17%	4.5	2.5	39
Oriental style chicken, 1 pkg	230	28%	7	2	25
Sirloin beef tips & mushroom sauce, 1 pkg	270	19%	6	2	31
Spaghetti w/meat sauce, 1 pkg	220	16%	3.5	1	31
Lean Cuisine—Café Classics					
Beef portobello, 1 pkg	210	21%	5	2.5	23
Chicken w/almonds, 1 pkg	260	15%	4.5	0.5	35
Chicken carbonara, 1 pkg	270	19%	6	2	32
Chicken fried rice, 1 pkg	280	18%	6	1	36
Fiesta grilled chicken, 1 pkg	250	24%	7	3	24
Garlic beef & broccoli, 1 pkg	170	29%	6	2	10
Shrimp & angel hair, 1 pkg	240	17%	4.5	1	32
Sweet & sour chicken, 1 pkg	300	8%	3	0.5	50
Teriyaki steak, 1 pkg	280	18%	6	2	34
Three cheese chicken, 1 pkg	230	39%	10	3	12
Three cheese stuffed rigatoni, 1 pkg	240	21%	6	3	31

Product and Portion Size	Calories	% Cal from Fat	Total Fat (g)	Bad Fat (g)	Net Carbs (g)
Lean Cuisine—Comfort Classics					
Baked chicken, 1 pkg	240	17%	4.5	1	31
Baked lemon pepper fish, 1 pkg	230	22%	6	2	21
Beef pot roast, 1 pkg	190	26%	6	1.5	19
Beef peppercorn, 1 pkg	220	27%	7	2.5	22
Cheese lasagna w/chicken scaloppini, 1 pkg	280	25%	2	0	29
Honey roasted pork, 1 pkg	230	35%	9	3.5	13
Meatloaf & whipped potatoes, 1 pkg	250	24%	7	2.5	24
Roast turkey & vegetables, 1 pkg	150	30%	5	1	9
Salisbury steak, 1 pkg	280	29%	9	4.5	22
Southern beef tips, 1 pkg	250	18%	5	2	33
Lean Cuisine—Dinnertime Selects					
Chicken Florentine, 1 pkg	390	18%	8	2.5	49
Chicken portobello, 1 pkg	380	16%	7	2	51
Grilled chicken & penne pasta, 1 pkg	330	12%	4.5	1.5	46
Jumbo rigatoni w/meatballs, 1 pkg	390	18%	8	2.5	49
Lemon garlic shrimp, 1 pkg	280	21%	7	3.5	31
Orange peel chicken, 1 pkg	400	23%	10	1.5	46

Product and Portion Size	Calories	% Cal from Fat	Total Fat (g)	Bad Fat (g)	Net Carbs (g)
Lean Cuisine—One Dish Favorites					
Asian style pot stickers, 1 pkg	320	19%	6	2	52
Cheese ravioli, 1 pkg	250	20%	6	3.5	33
Chicken chow mein w/rice	190	13%	2.5	0.5	27
Chicken enchilada suiza, 1 pkg	270	15%	4.5	2	44
Four cheese cannelloni, 1 pkg	240	25%	7	3.5	23
Macaroni & beef, 1 pkg	250	18%	5	2	32
Mandarin chicken, 1 pkg	240	13%	4	1	34
Santa Fe style rice & beans, 1 pkg	290	17%	6	2.5	44
Stuffed cabbage w/whipped potatoes, 1 pkg	200	25%	6	1.5	21
Swedish meatballs w/pasta, 1 pkg	280	21%	7	3	30
Three bean chili w/rice, 1 pkg	270	22%	7	2	36
Vegetable eggroll, 1 pkg	310	15%	5	1	57
Lean Cuisine—Skillets					
Asian style chicken & vegetables, 1 pkg	160	16%	2.5	0.5	20
Chicken alfredo, 1 pkg	190	21%	4.5	2	22
Chicken primavera, 1 pkg	180	14%	2.5	0.5	27
Chicken teriyaki, 1 pkg	230	9%	2	1	36

Product and Portion Size	Calories	% Cal from Fat	Total Fat (g)	Bad Fat (g)	Net Carbs (g)
Garlic chicken, 1 pkg	240	15%	4	2	37
Herb chicken, 1 pkg	160	19%	3.5	1	18
Roasted turkey, 1 pkg	130	12%	1.5	0.5	20
Three cheese chicken, 1 pkg	200	22%	5	2	22
Lean Cuisine—Spa Cuisine					
Chicken Mediterranean, 1 pkg	220	16%	4	0.5	27
Chicken in peanut sauce, 1 pkg	280	25%	8	1.5	37
Oven roasted beef burgundy, 1 pkg	300	20%	7	3	40
Pork w/cherry sauce, 1 pkg	260	13%	4	1.5	37
Rosemary chicken, 1 pkg	220	16%	4	2	26
Salmon w/basil, 1 pkg	230	19%	6	2	20
Salmon w/lemon dill sauce, 1 pkg	240	21%	6	2.5	26
On-Cor					
Chicken & dumplings, 1 cup	170	41%	8	3	17
Chicken parmesan, 1 patty + ¼ cup sauce	260	50%	14	4.3	15
Macaroni & cheese, 1 cup	170	15%	3	2	23
Salisbury steak & gravy, 1 patty + ⅓ cup gravy	200	60%	13	7	7
Stuffed green pepper, 1 pepper + ¼ cup sauce	230	57%	14	7	19

Product and Portion Size	Calories	% Cal from Fat	Total Fat (g)	Bad Fat (g)	Net Carbs (g)
Stouffer's—Corner Bistro					
Chicken carbonara, 1 pkg	530	36%	22	12	46
Garlic chicken pasta, 1 pkg	340	21%	8	2	38
Grilled chicken rosemary, 1 pkg	420	36%	17	5	38
Philly style steak & cheese panini, 1 pkg	340	41%	16	6	30
Seafood scampi, 1 pkg	410	24%	11	5	51
Southwestern style chicken panini, 1 pkg	360	42%	16	7	28
Stouffer's—Dinners					
Chicken fettuccini, 1 pkg	620	35%	24	6	62
Meatloaf, 1 pkg	560	46%	29	13.5	32
Roast turkey breast, 1 pkg	390	31%	13	3.5	42
Slow roast beef, 1 pkg	320	44%	15	4.5	22
Stouffer's—Entrees & Grilled Entrees					
Chicken ala king, 1 pkg	410	31%	14	4	51
Fried chicken breast, 1 pkg	360	44%	18	4.5	28
Grilled chicken teriyaki, 1 pkg	300	10%	3.5	1	42
Grilled herb chicken, 1 pkg	250	20%	6	1	26
Grilled lemon pepper chicken, 1 pkg	260	24%	7	2	22

Product and Portion Size	Calories	% Cal from Fat	Total Fat (g)	Bad Fat (g)	Net Carbs (g)
Stouffer's—Skillets					
Chicken alfredo, ½ pkg	410	24%	11	5	47
Chicken & pasta, ½ pkg	340	18%	7	2	36
Homestyle beef, ½ pkg	300	33%	11	3	26
Teriyaki chicken, ½ pkg	310	13%	4.5	1	38
Weight Watchers—Smart Ones					
Angel hair marinara, 1 pkg	230	7%	1.5	0.5	39
Broccoli & cheddar roasted potatoes, 1 pkg	220	23%	6	3	29
Chicken carbonara, 1 pkg	250	16%	4.5	1.5	20
Chicken fettucini, 1 pkg	340	21%	8	4	38
Chicken Mirabella, 1 pkg	150	11%	2	0.5	30
Chicken parmesan, 1 pkg	290	17%	5	1.5	31
Creamy rigatoni w/broccoli & chicken, 1 pkg	290	28%	8	3	31
Dragon shrimp lo mein, 1 pkg	240	15%	4	1	33
Fajita chicken supreme, 1 pkg	260	23%	7	3	28
Golden baked garlic chicken, 1 pkg	270	19%	5	1	40
Honey Dijon chicken, 1 pkg	220	14%	3.5	0.5	36
Lasagna Florentine, 1 pkg	290	28%	9	5	36

Product and Portion Size	Calories	% Cal from Fat	Total Fat (g)	Bad Fat (g)	Net Carbs (g)
Meatloaf w/gravy, 1 pkg	260	31%	8	2.5	17
Penne pollo, 1 pkg	280	14%	6	2.5	36
Peppersteak, 1 pkg	250	16%	4.5	1.5	33
Radiatore romano, 1 pkg	290	24%	7	3	39
Ravioli Florentine, 1 pkg	250	18%	5	2	36
Roast beef w/gravy, 1 pkg	210	38%	9	3	17
Salisbury steak, 1 pkg	260	23%	7	3	23
Santa Fe style rice and beans, 1 pkg	310	23%	7	3	47
Shrimp marinara, 1 pkg	180	8%	1.5	0	27
Slow roasted turkey breast, 1 pkg	210	29%	7	2	16
Southwest style adobe chicken, 1 pkg	310	29%	10	3	33
Swedish meatballs, 1 pkg	270	17%	5	2	32
Thai chicken & rice noodles, 1 pkg	260	13%	4	0.5	41
Three cheese ziti marinara, 1 pkg	290	21%	7	2.5	35
Tuna noodle gratin, 1 pkg	250	16%	4.5	1.5	35
FROZEN SANDWICHES/POCKETS					
Amy's Kitchen					
Broccoli & cheese in a pocket sandwich, 1	270	33%	10	4	34

Product and Portion Size	Calories	% Cal from Fat	Total Fat (g)	Bad Fat (g)	Net Carbs (g)
Cheese pizza in a pocket sandwich, 1	300	27%	9	3.5	38
Roasted vegetable in a pocket sandwich, 1	230	30%	8	1.5	31
Soy cheese pizza in a pocket sandwich, 1	260	27%	8	0.5	38
Spinach feta in a pocket sandwich, 1	260	31%	9	4.5	31
Spinach pizza in a pocket sandwich, 1	280	29%	9	4	34
Tofu scramble in a pocket sandwich, 1	180	28%	6	0	22
Vegetable pie in a pocket sandwich, 1	300	27%	9	1.5	42
Croissant Pockets					
Chicken alfredo, 1	320	44%	15	7	35
Egg, sausage, cheese, 1	360	50%	20	7	34
Ham & cheese, 1	340	41%	16	8	33
Pepperoni pizza, 1	390	46%	20	10	39
Philly cheese steak, 1	360	50%	19	8	33
Hot Pockets					
3 cheese & chicken quesadilla, 1 pc	320	38%	13	6	38
4 cheese pizza, 1 pc	390	46%	20	7	41
4 meat & 4 cheese, 1 pc	300	57%	19	8	35
Beef taco, 1 pc	320	38%	13	6	37
Cheeseburger, 1 pc	340	35%	14	6	40

Product and Portion Size	Calories	% Cal from Fat	Total Fat (g)	Bad Fat (g)	Net Carbs (g)
Chicken fajita, 1 pc	290	34%	11	4	36
Ham & cheese, 1 pc	310	39%	13	5	33
Italian 3 meat pizza, 1 pc	350	40%	16	6	39
Meatballs & mozzarella, 1 pc	330	36%	14	5	39
Sausage pizza, 1 pc	360	47%	19	7	37
Supreme pizza, 1 pc	380	47%	20	8	38
Lean Pockets					
Cheeseburger, 1 pc	280	23%	7	4	40
Chicken parmesan, 1 pc	280	21%	7	3	41
Five cheese pizza, 1 pc	390	46%	20	7.5	37
Meatball & mozzarella, 1 pc	290	21%	7	3.5	42
Philly steak & cheese, 1 pc	280	21%	7	3.5	38
Sausage, egg & cheese, 1 pc	140	29%	4.5	1.5	17
Sausage & pepperoni, 1 pc	280	21%	7	3.5	39
Turkey, broccoli & cheese, 1 pc	270	22%	7	3.5	37
Lightlife					
Tortilla wrap, Mexican, 1	340	19%	7	1	44
Tortilla wrap, ranchero, 1	300	18%	6	1	41

Product and Portion Size	Calories	% Cal from Fat	Total Fat (g)	Bad Fat (g)	Net Carbs (g)
Smart Ones—Smartwich					
Garden veggies & mozzarella, 1	270	19%	6	2.5	37
Ham & cheddar 1	270	22%	6	3	39
Pepperoni pizza, 1	290	21%	7	3.5	39
Three cheese & Italian meatball, 1	290	21%	7	2.5	40
FRUIT SNACKS					
Betty Crocker Fruit by the Foot, all flavors, 1 roll	80	13%	1	0	17
Betty Crocker Fruit Roll Ups, all flavors, 1 roll	50	10%	1	0	12
Betty Crocker Fruit Flavored Shapes, 1 pouch	80	0%	0	0	21
GARLIC, raw, 1 oz	42	2%	0	0	8
GELATIN					
Jell-O, all flavors, regular, ½ cup prep.	80	0%	0	0	19
Jell-O, all flavors, sugar free, ½ cup prep.	10	0%	0	0	0
Royal, all flavors, regular, ½ cup prep.	70	0%	0	0	17
Royal, all flavors, sugar free, ½ cup prep.	5	0%	0	0	0
GRAPES, green or red, 1½ cup	90	10%	1	0	23
GRAPE JUICE/DRINK					
Capri Sun, juice drink, 8 oz	100	0%	0	0	25

Product and Portion Size	Calories	% Cal from Fat	Total Fat (g)	Bad Fat (g)	Net Carbs (g)
Cascadian Farms, organic grape juice, 8 oz	150	0%	0	0	38
Kool-Aid, sugar-sweetened, 8 oz	60	0%	0	0	16
Kool-Aid, sugar-free, 1g	5	0%	0	0	0
Welch's, light w/calcium, 8 oz	70	0%	0	0	18
Welch's, purple 100% juice, 8 oz	170	0%	0	0	42
Welch's, white 100% juice, 8 oz	160	0%	0	0	39
Welch's, white grape peach, 8 oz	160	0%	0	0	89
GRAPEFRUIT					
Fresh, pink or red, ½ fruit	52	2%	0	0	11
Fresh, white, ½ fruit	39	3%	0	0	9
Del Monte, sections, red, ½ cup	90	0%	0	0	11
Del Monte, sun fresh red, ½ cup	80	0%	0	0	17
Del Monte, sun fresh white in real juice ½ cup	45	0%	0	0	7
Fruit Naturals, red grapefruit, ½ cup	60	0%	0	0	15
GRAPEFRUIT JUICE					
Dole, ruby red 100% juice blend, 11.5 oz	190	0%	0	0	47
Knudsen, organic, 8 oz	100	0%	0	0	23
Knudsen, rio red, 8 oz	140	0%	0	0	35

Product and Portion Size	Calories	% Cal from Fat	Total Fat (g)	Bad Fat (g)	Net Carbs (g)
Minute Maid, 100% juice, frozen, w/calcium, 8 oz	100	0%	0	0	25
Tropicana, 100% juice, ruby red, 8 oz	90	0%	0	0	22
Tropicana, sweet grapefruit, 8 oz	130	0%	0	0	31
GRAVY					
Boston Market, pan style beef, 2 oz	40	63%	2.5	1	3
Boston Market, pan style poultry, 2 oz	40	50%	2	1	3
Campbell's					
Beef, ¼ cup	25	36%	1	0.5	3
Brown w/onions, ¼ cup	25	36%	1	0	4
Chicken giblet, ¼ cup	30	45%	1.5	0.5	3
Chicken, ¼ cup	40	68%	3	1	3
Country style cream, ¼ cup	45	60%	3	1	3
Creamy mushroom, ¼ cup	20	23%	0.5	0.5	4
Fat free beef, ¼ cup	15	0%	0	0	3
Fat free chicken, ¼ cup	15	0%	0	0	3
Golden pork, ¼ cup	45	60%	3	1.5	3
Mushroom, ¼ cup	20	45%	1	0	3
Turkey, ¼ cup	25	36%	1	0.5	3

Product and Portion Size	Calories	% Cal from Fat	Total Fat (g)	Bad Fat (g)	Net Carbs (g)
Franco-American, beef, ¼ cup	25	36%	1	0.5	3
Franco-American, turkey, ¼ cup	25	36%	1	0.5	3
Franco-American, f-f slow roast beef, ¼ cup	20	0%	0	0	3
Franco-American, f-f slow roast chicken, ¼ cup	20	0%	0	0	4
Heinz, classic chicken, ¼ cup	25	40%	1	0	4
GREEN BEANS					
Fresh, boiled, no salt, 1 cup	44	7%	0	0	6
Canned					
Del Monte, cut, ½ cup	20	0%	0	0	2
Del Monte, cut Italian, ½ cup	30	0%	0	0	3
Del Monte, cut w/potatoes w/ham style, ½ cup	30	0%	0	0	5
Del Monte, French style, ½ cup	20	0%	0	0	2
Del Monte, seasoned, ½ cup	20	0%	0	0	2
S&W, cut, ½ cup	20	0%	0	0	2
S&W, cut green & wax beans, ½ cup	20	0%	0	0	2
S&W, dilled green, ½ cup	20	0%	0	0	4
Frozen					
Cascadian Farms, cut, organic, ¾ cup	30	0%	0	0	4

Product and Portion Size	Calories	% Cal from Fat	Total Fat (g)	Bad Fat (g)	Net Carbs (g)
Cascadian Farms, French w/almonds, ⅔ cup	70	43%	3	0	6
Green Giant, cut, ½ cup	20	0%	0	0	3
Green Giant, cut, low sodium, ½ cup	20	0%	0	0	3
Green Giant, French, ½ cup	20	0%	0	0	3
Green Giant, select whole, 1 cup	20	0%	0	0	2
Green Giant, green bean casserole, ⅔ cup	110	64%	8	3.5	7
Green Giant, green bean & garlic butter, ½ cup	50	20%	1	1	6
HADDOCK, baked, 3 oz	95	7%	1	0	0
HALIBUT, Atlantic & Pacific, baked, 3 oz	**119**	**19%**	**2**	**0**	**0**
Greenland, baked, 3 oz	203	67%	15	3	0
HAM					
Cured, extra lean, roasted, 3 oz	123	34%	5	2	1
Cured, regular, 3 oz	151	46%	8	3	0
Fresh, leg, shank, lean & fat, roasted, 3 oz	246	63%	17	6	0
Fresh, rump, lean & fat, roasted, 3 oz	214	51%	12	4	0
Healthy Choice, smoked ham, 2 oz	60	25%	1.5	0.5	2
Healthy Choice, Virginia brand, 2 oz	60	25%	1.5	0.5	2
Oscar Mayer, deli style, honey shaved, ⅕ pkg	50	20%	1	0.5	2
Oscar Mayer, smoked shaved, ⅕ pkg	45	22%	1	0	0

Product and Portion Size	Calories	% Cal from Fat	Total Fat (g)	Bad Fat (g)	Net Carbs (g)
HAMBURGER MIX (mix only)					
Bacon cheeseburger, ½ cup	190	26%	6	4	29
Beef pasta, ⅓ cup	110	5%	1	0	21
Beef taco, ½ cup	140	11%	1.5	0	27
Cheeseburger macaroni, ⅓ cup	160	13%	2.5	1	30
Cheesy enchilada, ½ cup	190	18%	4	2	35
Cheesy Italian shells, ½ cup	150	7%	1	0.5	31
Chili macaroni, ⅓ cup	130	8%	1	0	27
Double cheese pizza, ½ cup	150	10%	1.5	0.5	31
Italian sausage, ⅓ cup	140	11%	1.5	0.5	25
Lasagna, ⅔ cup	120	4%	0.5	0	25
Philly cheesesteak, ½ cup	150	33%	5	3	21
Ravioli & cheese, ½ cup	150	7%	1.5	0.5	30
Rice oriental, ¼ cup	140	4%	0.5	0	31
Salisbury, ⅔ cup	120	8%	1	0.5	23
Stroganoff, ⅔ cup	130	19%	2.5	2	22
Tomato basil penne, ⅓ cup	150	7%	1	0	29
Zesty Italian, ⅓ cup	140	7%	1	0	29

Product and Portion Size	Calories	% Cal from Fat	Total Fat (g)	Bad Fat (g)	Net Carbs (g)
HEALTH BARS AND SHAKES					
Atkins Advantage					
Almond brownie bar, 1	220	36%	9	4	15
Café mocha shake, 1 can	160	51%	9	1.5	2
Caramel chocolate peanut nougat bar, 1	150	40%	7	3.5	8
Caramel fudge brownie bar, 1	160	44%	8	5	8
Chocolate coconut bar, 1	230	39%	10	8	13
Chocolate delight shake, 1 can	170	47%	9	2	1
Chocolate peanut butter bar, 1	240	42%	11	6	12
Chocolate royale shake, 1 can	170	47%	9	2	2
Creamy vanilla shake, 1 can	170	47%	9	1.5	1
Golden oats granola bar, 1	210	33%	8	3.5	11
Strawberry supreme shake, 1 can	170	47%	9	1.5	2
Vanilla caramel crème shake, 1 can	170	47%	9	1.5	2
Atkins Morning Start					
Apple crisp bar, 1	180	44%	9	4.5	7
Chocolate chip bar, 1	160	38%	7	3.5	10
Creamy cinnamon bun bar, 1	150	40%	7	5	6

Product and Portion Size	Calories	% Cal from Fat	Total Fat (g)	Bad Fat (g)	Net Carbs (g)
Mixed berry bar, 1	150	33%	5	1	9
Oatmeal raisin bar, 1	140	32%	4	1	10
Strawberry crisp bar, 1	160	50%	9	4.5	7
Balance Bars					
Almond brownie, original, 1	200	30%	6	1.5	21
Caramel & chocolate, Carbwell, 1	190	32%	7	4	22
Chewy chocolate chip, Gold, 1	210	29%	7	4	21
Chocolate, original 1	200	25%	6	3.5	21
Chocolate fudge, Carbwell, 1	190	32%	6	4	21
Chocolate peanut butter, Carbwell, 1	200	35%	8	4	21
Chocolate peanut butter, Gold, 1	210	29%	7	4	21
Cookie dough, original 1	200	30%	6	3.5	21
Mocha chip, original, 1	200	25%	6	3.5	22
Rocky road, Gold, 1	210	29%	7	4	21
Yogurt honey peanut, original, 1	200	30%	6	3	21
Clif Bar					
Banana nut bread, 1	250	20%	6	1	38
Carrot cake, 1	240	15%	4	1.5	41

Product and Portion Size	Calories	% Cal from Fat	Total Fat (g)	Bad Fat (g)	Net Carbs (g)
Chocolate chip, 1	250	18%	5	2	40
Crunch peanut butter, 1	250	20%	6	1.5	35
Lemon poppyseed, 1	240	13%	3.5	1.5	41
Oatmeal raisin walnut, 1	240	19%	5	1	38
Luna					
Caramel nut brownie, 1	190	28%	6	3	23
Cherry covered chocolate, 1	180	25%	5	3	25
Chocolate peppermint stick, 1	180	25%	5	3	26
Cookies & cream delight, 1	180	22%	4.5	3	25
Key lime pie, 1	180	19%	4	3	23
Lemon zest, 1	180	19%	4	3	23
Peanut butter cookie, 1	180	28%	6	3	22
S'mores, 1	180	25%	5	3	23
Strawberries 'n crème, Sunrise, 1	**180**	**19%**	**4**	**2**	**24**
Vanilla almond, Sunrise, 1	**180**	**22%**	**4.5**	**2**	**24**
PowerBar, Harvest Whole Grain					
Dipped double chocolate crisp, 1	250	18%	5	2.5	37
Dipped oatmeal raisin, 1	250	18%	5	2	37

Product and Portion Size	Calories	% Cal from Fat	Total Fat (g)	Bad Fat (g)	Net Carbs (g)
Heart healthy apple cinnamon crisp, 1	240	15%	4	0.5	37
Heart healthy strawberry crunch, 1	240	15%	4	0.5	37
PowerBar Performance					
Apple cinnamon, 1	230	11%	2.5	0.5	42
Banana, 1	230	9%	2.5	0.5	42
Chocolate peanut butter, 1	240	13%	3	1	42
Oatmeal raisin, 1	230	11%	2.5	0.5	42
Vanilla crisp, 1	230	11%	2.5	0.5	42
Wild berry, 1	230	11%	2.5	0.5	42
PowerBar Pria 110 Plus					
Chocolate peanut crunch, 1	110	27%	3.5	2	15
Double chocolate cookie, 1	110	23%	3	2.5	15
French vanilla crisp, 1	110	23%	3	2.5	16
Mint chocolate cookie, 1	110	27%	3.5	2.5	14
PowerBar Protein Plus					
Chocolate crisp, 1	290	17%	6	3.5	38
Chocolate peanut butter, 1	300	17%	6	3.5	38
Cookies & cream, 1	300	17%	6	3.5	37
Vanilla yogurt, 1	300	17%	6	3.5	37

Product and Portion Size	Calories	% Cal from Fat	Total Fat (g)	Bad Fat (g)	Net Carbs (g)
PowerBar Triple Threat					
Caramel peanut fusion, 1	230	30%	8	4.5	26
Caramel peanut crisp, 1	220	20%	5	2	28
Chocolate caramel, 1	230	30%	8	4.5	26
Chocolate peanut butter crisp, 1	220	20%	5	2	28
Slim Fast Optima Meal Bars					
Blueberry crisp, 1	180	19%	4	2.5	25
Chocolate chip granola, 1	220	23%	6	3.5	33
Milk chocolate peanut, 1	220	20%	5	3	33
Oatmeal raisin, 1	220	20%	5	3	33
Peanut butter chewy granola, 1	220	23%	6	3	33
Rich chocolate brownie, 1	220	20%	5	3.5	32
Strawberry cheesecake, 1	220	23%	6	4	32
Trail mix chewy granola, 1	210	21%	5	1	32
Slim Fast Optima Shakes					
Cappuccino delight, 1 can	180	28%	6	2	20
Creamy milk chocolate, 1 can	190	26%	6	2.5	20
French vanilla, 1 can	190	26%	6	2.5	19

Product and Portion Size	Calories	% Cal from Fat	Total Fat (g)	Bad Fat (g)	Net Carbs (g)
Rich chocolate royale, 1 can	180	25%	5	2	18
Strawberry 'n cream, 1 can	180	25%	5	2	18
Slim Fast Optima Snack Bars					
Apple cinnamon muffin, 1	140	36%	5	0.5	20
Banana & nut muffin, 1	150	47%	8	0.5	17
Blueberry muffin, 1	140	36%	5	0.5	21
Chocolate mint crisp, 1	120	33%	4	3	18
Chocolate peanut nougat, 1	120	29%	4	.5	19
Crispy peanut caramel, 1	120	29%	4	3	1
Oatmeal raisin cookie, 1	120	25%	3.5	1.5	18
Peanut butter crunch, 1	120	29%	4	2	20
HERRING, Atlantic, kippered, 1 oz	**61**	**51%**	**3**	**1**	**3**
Atlantic, pickled, 1 oz	**74**	**62%**	**5**	**1**	**3**
Pacific, broiled, 3 oz	**212**	**64%**	**15**	**4**	**0**
HONEY, 1 Tbs	64	0%	0	0	17
HONEYDEW, raw, balls, 1 cup	64	3%	0	0	15
HORSERADISH, prep., 1 Tbs	7	12%	0	0	2
Woeber's, sauce, 1 tsp	20	75%	1.5	0	27

Product and Portion Size	Calories	% Cal from Fat	Total Fat (g)	Bad Fat (g)	Net Carbs (g)
HUMMUS					
Athenos, artichoke & garlic, 1 oz	45	44%	2.5	0	3
Athenos, black olive, 1 oz	50	50%	3	0	4
Athenos, cucumber dill, 1 oz	50	50%	3	0	4
Athenos, original, 1 oz	50	50%	3	0	4
Athenos, roasted eggplant, 1 oz	45	44%	2	0	4
Athenos, roasted garlic, 1 oz	50	50%	3	0	4
Athenos, roasted red pepper, 1 oz	50	60%	3	0	4
Fantastic Foods, 2 Tbs	60	33%	2	0	5
ICE CREAM					
Ben & Jerry's					
Black & tan, ½ cup	230	52%	13	9	23
Butter pecan, ½ cup	280	68%	21	10	31
Cherry Garcia, ½ cup	250	52%	14	10	20
Chocolate, ½ cup	260	54%	16	11	23
Chunky monkey, ½ cup	300	53%	18	10	29
Coffee, ½ cup	240	58%	15	10	21
Fossil fuel, ½ cup	280	54%	18	12	30

Product and Portion Size	Calories	% Cal from Fat	Total Fat (g)	Bad Fat (g)	Net Carbs (g)
Half-baked, ½ cup	280	43%	14	9	33
Mint chocolate cookie, ½ cup	260	54%	16	9	26
NY Super fudge chunk, ½ cup	310	58%	20	11	27
Neapolitan dynamite, ½ cup	250	48%	13	9	28
Turtle soup, ½ cup	280	50%	15	10	29
Vanilla Heath bar crunch, ½ cup	290	55%	18	12	29
Vermonty python, ½ cup	310	55%	19	11	29
Breyers					
Butter almond, ½ cup	160	56%	10	4.5	15
Butter pecan, ½ cup	160	56%	10	4.5	14
Caramel fudge, ½ cup	160	44%	7	4.5	20
Caramel praline, ½ cup	170	35%	7	4	22
Cherry vanilla, ½ cup	140	43%	6	4	17
Chocolate, ½ cup	140	50%	8	4.5	17
Chocolate chip, natural, ½ cup	160	50%	8	6	17
Chocolate chip cookie dough, ½ cup	160	44%	8	5	20
Cookies & cream, natural, ½ cup	160	44%	8	5	19
French vanilla, ½ cup	140	50%	8	5	15

Product and Portion Size	Calories	% Cal from Fat	Total Fat (g)	Bad Fat (g)	Net Carbs (g)
Mint chocolate chip, natural, ½ cup	160	50%	8	5	17
Peach, ½ cup	120	38%	5	3	17
Rocky road, ½ cup	160	44%	8	4.5	19
Strawberry, ½ cup	120	42%	5	3.5	15
Vanilla fudge brownie, ½ cup	150	40%	7	4.5	20
Vanilla fudge twirl, ½ cup	130	46%	6	4	17
Breyers, Double Churned					
Chocolate caramel brownie, ½ cup	160	38%	7	4.5	22
Creamy chocolate, ½ cup	140	43%	7	4.5	17
Strawberries & cream, ½ cup	130	38%	6	3.5	16
Vanilla, chocolate, strawberry, ½ cup	140	43%	7	4.5	17
98% f-f vanilla, ½ cup	90	17%	1.5	1	19
Dreyer's—Grand					
Almond praline, ½ cup	150	40%	7	4	20
Butter pecan, ½ cup	170	53%	10	4.5	16
Chocolate, ½ cup	150	47%	8	4.5	16
Cookie dough, ½ cup	180	44%	9	6	21
Fudge tracks, ½ cup	180	56%	11	6	18

Product and Portion Size	Calories	% Cal from Fat	Total Fat (g)	Bad Fat (g)	Net Carbs (g)
Mocha almond fudge, ½ cup	160	50%	9	4.5	17
Peanut butter cup, ½ cup	180	50%	10	4	19
Rocky road, ½ cup	170	53%	10	5	19
Spumoni, ½ cup	150	47%	8	4.5	16
Toffee bar crunch, ½ cup	170	47%	9	5	19
Turtle sundae, ½ cup	160	50%	9	4.5	18
Dreyers—Slow-Churned Light					
Butter pecan, ½ cup	120	38%	5	2	16
Chocolate chip, ½ cup	120	38%	4.5	3	17
Cookies & cream, ½ cup	120	29%	4	2	18
Mint chocolate chip, ½ cup	120	33%	4.5	3	17
Neapolitan, ½ cup	100	25%	3	2	15
Peanut butter cup, ½ cup	130	38%	6	3	17
Rocky road, ½ cup	120	29%	4	2	17
Strawberry, ½ cup	110	23%	3	1.5	18
Vanilla bean, ½ cup	100	30%	3.5	2	15
Vanilla chocolate, ½ cup	100	30%	3.5	2	15

Product and Portion Size	Calories	% Cal from Fat	Total Fat (g)	Bad Fat (g)	Net Carbs (g)
Haagen-Dazs—Regular					
Bailey's Irish cream, ½ cup	270	56%	17	10.5	23
Banana split, ½ cup	280	50%	16	9	31
Black walnut, ½ cup	300	66%	22	11.5	21
Butter pecan, ½ cup	310	67%	23	11	21
Cherry vanilla, ½ cup	240	58%	15	9.5	23
Chocolate, ½ cup	270	59%	18	11.5	21
Chocolate peanut butter, ½ cup	360	61%	24	11	25
English toffee, ½ cup	350	57%	22	13.5	33
Rocky road, ½ cup	300	53%	18	9	28
Strawberry cheesecake, ½ cup	260	54%	15	8.5	27
Vanilla fudge brownie, ½ cup	300	57%	19	11	28
Haagen-Dazs—Light					
Blueberry cheesecake, ½ cup	230	26%	7	4	36
Cherry fudge truffle, ½ cup	230	26%	7	4	37
Cookies & cream, ½ cup	210	24%	6	3.5	33
Mint chip, ½ cup	230	30%	8	5	34
Vanilla caramel brownie, ½ cup	240	25%	7	4	37

Product and Portion Size	Calories	% Cal from Fat	Total Fat (g)	Bad Fat (g)	Net Carbs (g)
ICE CREAM NOVELTIES					
Dreyer's					
Dibs, caramel w/chocolate coating, 26 pcs	440	66%	32	22	35
Dibs, cookies & cream w/chocolate coat, 26 pcs	410	63%	29	29	33
Dibs, peanut butter w/chocolate coat, 26 pcs	510	69%	39	23	32
Dibs, vanilla w/chocolate coat, 26 pcs	420	69%	32	19	29
Dibs, vanilla w/Nestle Crunch, 26 pcs	380	66%	28	20	29
Fruit bars: creamy coconut, 1	130	19%	3	2.5	22
Fruit bars: grape, 1	80	0%	0	0	20
Fruit bars: orange & cream, 1	80	19%	1.5	0.5	16
Fruit bars: strawberry, 1	80	0%	0	0	21
Good Humor					
Chocolate éclair bar, 1	160	44%	8	3.5	20
Cone, Oreo cookies & cream, 1	220	41%	10	6	31
Cone, premium sundae, 1	260	54%	15	9	28
Cone, vanilla king, 1	250	48%	13	8	29
Cyclone caramel tracks, 1	500	42%	23	16.5	66
Cyclone chocolate chip cookie dough, 1	570	46%	29	18.5	72

Product and Portion Size	Calories	% Cal from Fat	Total Fat (g)	Bad Fat (g)	Net Carbs (g)
Cyclone cookies & cream, 1	540	46%	28	15	66
Strawberry shortcake bar, 1	170	47%	9	4.5	21
Toasted almond bar, 1	180	50%	10	4.5	21
Haagen-Dazs					
Brownie bar, 1	360	61%	24	13	29
Chocolate & dark chocolate bar, 1	300	63%	21	13	23
Coffee & almond crunch, 1	310	65%	22	12	22
Mint & dark chocolate, 1	290	62%	20	12	22
Vanilla & milk chocolate, 1	290	66%	21	14	22
Klondike					
Bar, chocolate, 1	250	64%	17	13	21
Bar, Heath, 1	270	63%	19	13.5	24
Bar, Krunch, 1	250	60%	17	13	22
Bar, Oreo, 1	260	58%	17	12	26
Bar, Reese's, 1	270	59%	18	11	23
Bar, vanilla, 1	250	60%	17	13	22
Cone, vanilla, 1	280	50%	16	9	29
Cone, vanilla & vanilla fudge, 1	300	50%	16	10	34

Product and Portion Size	Calories	% Cal from Fat	Total Fat (g)	Bad Fat (g)	Net Carbs (g)
Sandwich, ice cream cookie, 1	260	38%	11	5	37
Sandwich, vanilla, 1	190	32%	7	4	29
Slim-A-Bear, cookies & cream, 1	110	9%	1	0	22
Slim-A-Bear, krunch, 1	170	53%	10	8	18
Slim-A-Bear, vanilla, 1	170	53%	9	8	17
Slim-A-Bear, vanilla sandwich, 1	130	8%	1.5	0	26
Popsicle					
Creamsicle, 1.65 oz	70	21%	1.5	1	12
Creamsicle, sugar free, 1	40	38%	2	1.5	10
Fudgsicle, 1.65 oz	60	25%	1.5	1.5	12
Tropicals, sugar free, 1	15	0%	0	0	4
ICE CREAM SUBSTITUTES (Non-Dairy)					
Soy Delicious—Organic					
Butter pecan, ½ cup	160	50%	7	1	19
Chocolate velvet, ½ cup	130	23%	3.5	0.5	22
Creamy vanilla, ½ cup	130	19%	3	0	21
Mocha fudge, ½ cup	130	19%	3	0	23
Peanut butter, ½ cup	150	33%	6	1	20

Product and Portion Size	Calories	% Cal from Fat	Total Fat (g)	Bad Fat (g)	Net Carbs (g)
Soy Delicious—Novelties					
Li'l Buddies, chocolate, 1	150	27%	4.5	2	22
Li'l Buddies, vanilla, 1	180	22%	4.5	2	25
So Delicious Dairy-Free bars, orange, 1	80	12%	1.5	0	16
So Delicious Dairy-Free bars, fudge, 1	80	25%	2	0	16
Sweet Nothings, fudge bar, 1	100	0%	0	0	23
Sweet Nothings, mango raspberry, 1	100	0%	0	0	23
Tofutti					
Better pecan, ½ cup	210	58%	13	2	22
Chocolate fudge, low-fat, ½ cup	145	25%	4	1	25
Chocolate cookie crunch, ½ cup	190	53%	11	2	26
Chocolate supreme, ½ cup	180	56%	11	2	18
Coffee marshmallow swirl, low-fat, ½ cup	120	23%	4	1	25
Vanilla, ½ cup	190	50%	11	2	20
Vanilla fudge, ½ cup	190	43%	9	2	25
Tofutti Cheesecake Supreme, chocolate, blueberry, or strawberry, ½ cup	200	52%	12	2	20

Product and Portion Size	Calories	% Cal from Fat	Total Fat (g)	Bad Fat (g)	Net Carbs (g)
Tofutti—Cuties					
Chocolate	130	35%	5	1	16
Coffee break, ½ cup	130	35%	5	1	16
Cookies & cream, ½ cup	120	45%	6	1	17
Peanut butter, ½ cup	165	44%	8	2	20
Totally vanilla, ½ cup	120	38%	5	1	16
Vanilla, ½ cup	120	38%	5	1	17
Tofutti Super Soy, Bella vanilla, ½ cup	160	45%	8	0	20
Tofutti Super Soy, NY chocolate, ½ cup	170	48%	9	0	22
JAM, JELLY, PRESERVES					
Cascadian Farm Fruit Spreads, organic					
Apricot, concord grape, or strawberry, 1 Tbs	40	0%	0	0	10
Blackberry, blueberry, or raspberry, 1 Tbs	45	0%	0	0	11
Smucker's jam: concord grape, 1 Tbs	50	0%	0	0	12
Smucker's jam, red plum, 1 Tbs	50	0%	0	0	13
Smucker's jelly, all flavors, 1 Tbs	50	0%	0	0	13
Smucker's Simply Fruit, all, 1 Tbs	40	0%	0	0	10
Welch's grape jelly, 1 Tbs	50	0%	0	0	13
Welch's jam, marmalade, 1 Tbs	50	0%	0	0	13

Product and Portion Size	Calories	% Cal from Fat	Total Fat (g)	Bad Fat (g)	Net Carbs (g)
KALE, fresh, cooked, no salt, chopped, 1 cup	**36**	**12%**	**1**	**0**	**4**
KETCHUP					
Del Monte, 1 Tbs	15	0%	0	0	4
Hunts, 1 Tbs	15	0%	0	0	4
KIELBASA					
Hillshire, Polska, 2 oz	180	78%	15	6	2
Hillshire, turkey, 2 oz	90	50%	5	2	2
Jennie-O, turkey, 2 oz	70	36%	3	1	1
KNOCKWURST, Hebrew National beef, 1 link	260	85%	24	11	1
KUMQUAT, raw, 1	13	10%	0	0	2
LAMB					
Australian, sirloin chop, lean, broiled, 3 oz	160	37%	7	3	0
Australian, leg, whole, lean, roasted, 3 oz	162	38%	7	3	0
Australian shoulder blade, lean & fat, broiled, 3 oz	247	68%	19	9	0
Domestic, leg, sirloin half, lean & fat, 3 oz	241	62%	17	7	0
Domestic, loin, lean, roasted, 3 oz	172	44%	8	3	0
Domestic, rib, lean & fat, roasted, 3 oz	290	73%	23	10	0
NZ, frozen, loin, lean & fat, broiled, 3 oz	252	65%	18	9	0

Product and Portion Size	Calories	% Cal from Fat	Total Fat (g)	Bad Fat (g)	Net Carbs (g)
NZ, frozen, rib, lean, roasted, 3 oz	167	47%	9	4	0
NZ, frozen, shoulder, lean & fat, braised, 3 oz	291	63%	20	10	0
LEMON, raw, peeled, 1 cup	61	9%	1	0	20
LEMONADE					
Country Time, reg & pink, 8 oz	60	0%	0	0	16
Country Time, strawberry, 8 oz	80	0%	0	0	20
Crystal Light, sugar free, 8 oz	5	0%	0	0	0
Kool-Aid, sugar sweetened, 8 oz	70	0%	0	0	17
Kool-Aid, unsweetened, 8 oz	0	0%	0	0	0
Minute Maid (carton), 8 oz	110	0%	0	0	31
Minute Maid (frozen) country style, 8 oz	110	0%	0	0	29
Minute Maid (carton), raspberry lemonade, 8 oz	120	0%	0	0	32
Newman's Own old fashioned roadside, 8 oz	110	0%	0	0	27
LENTILS, cooked, no salt, 1 cup	230	3%	1	0	24
LETTUCE					
Butterhead (Boston, bibb), 1 cup shredded	7	14%	0	0	1
Green leaf, 1 cup shredded	5	3%	0	0	1
Iceberg, 1 cup shredded	8	8%	0	0	2

Product and Portion Size	Calories	% Cal from Fat	Total Fat (g)	Bad Fat (g)	Net Carbs (g)
Red leaf, 1 cup shredded	4	12%	0	0	1
Romaine, 1 cup shredded	8	15%	0	0	2
LIMA BEANS, fresh, boiled, no salt, 1 cup	209	2%	10	0	31
Birds Eye, baby limas (frozen), ½ cup	110	0%	0	0	15
Birds Eye, Fordhook (frozen), ½ cup	100	0%	0	0	14
Del Monte, canned, ½ cup	80	0%	0	0	11
Green Giant, baby limas (frozen), ½ cup	80	0%	0	0	12
Green Giant, baby limas & butter, ⅔ cup	110	14%	1.5	1	16
LIME, fresh, 1 fruit	20	5%	0	0	5
LIVER (see beef, chicken)					
LIVERWURST, Oscar Mayer Braunschweiger, 2 oz	190	79%	17	6	1
LOBSTER					
Northern, cooked, 3 oz	83	6%	1	0	1
Spiny, cooked, 3 oz	122	12%	2	0	3
LUNCHABLES					
Bologna & American cracker stackers, 1 pkg	390	51%	22	10	38
Chicken dunks, 1 pkg	300	15%	5	1	51
Chicken shakeups, BBQ, 1 pkg	210	24%	6	2	27

Product and Portion Size	Calories	% Cal from Fat	Total Fat (g)	Bad Fat (g)	Net Carbs (g)
Chicken strips, maxed out, 1 pkg	480	27%	15	4.5	72
Ham & American cracker stackers, 1 pkg	420	36%	17	9.5	53
Ham & cheese cracker stackers, 1 pkg	400	45%	20	10	39
Ham & Swiss, 1 pkg	340	47%	17	10	23
Ham & Swiss, low fat, cracker stackers, 1 pkg	340	24%	9	4	50
Mini burgers, grilled, 1 pkg	410	29%	14	9.5	55
Mini hot dogs, 1 pkg	400	28%	12	4	62
Nachos, 1 pkg	380	50%	21	6	40
Pepperoni pizza, 1 pkg	310	32%	11	4	34
Pizza cracker stackers, 1 pkg	420	38%	18	8.5	49
Pizza extra cheesy, 1 pkg	310	29%	10	4.5	34
Pizza stix, Maxed out, 1 pkg	680	13%	10	4.5	127
Pizza & Treatza, 1 pkg	460	20%	10	4.5	75
Sub sandwich, ham, turkey, cheddar, 1 pkg	460	39%	20	7.5	50
Taco beef, 1 pkg	460	24%	12	5	67
Turkey & American cracker stackers, 1 pkg	390	44%	19	10	38
Turkey & cheddar, 1 pkg	340	53%	20	10	22
Turkey & cheddar, cracker stackers, 1 pkg	380	29%	13	6.5	56
Turkey, ham, swiss, cheddar, 1 pkg	360	47%	19	10	25

Product and Portion Size	Calories	% Cal from Fat	Total Fat (g)	Bad Fat (g)	Net Carbs (g)
LUNCHEON LOAF					
Oscar Mayer, ham & cheese loaf, 1 oz	60	67%	4.5	2.5	1
Oscar Mayer, luncheon loaf spiced, 1 oz	60	67%	4.5	1.5	3
Oscar Mayer, olive loaf, 1 oz	80	75%	6	2	2
Oscar Mayer, pickle & pimento loaf, 1 oz	80	75%	6	2	2
MACADAMIA NUTS, dry roasted, no salt, 1 oz	**203**	**89%**	**21**	**3**	**2**
MACARONI (see "Pasta")					
MACARONI & CHEESE (boxed, mix.) (also see "Pasta" and "Frozen Dinners")					
Kraft Deluxe w/original cheddar cheese, 3.5 oz	320	28%	10	3.5	44
Kraft Deluxe sharp cheddar, 3.5 oz	320	28%	10	3.5	42
Kraft Dinner Deluxe ½ the fat, 2 oz	200	10%	2	1	36
Kraft Dinner Deluxe 4 cheese sauce, 3.5 oz	290	14%	4.5	2.5	48
Kraft Premium cheesy alfredo, 2 oz	260	8%	2.5	1	47
Kraft Premium thick N creamy, 2 oz	250	8%	2	1	48
Kraft Premium three cheese, 2 oz	260	8%	2.5	1	47
Kraft Rotini & white cheddar w/broccoli, 4.4 oz	390	36%	15	5	46
Kraft The Cheesiest, 2 oz	260	8%	2.5	1	47

Product and Portion Size	**Calories**	**% Cal from Fat**	**Total Fat (g)**	**Bad Fat (g)**	**Net Carbs (g)**
MACKEREL					
Atlantic, broiled, 3 oz	**223**	**61%**	**15**	**4**	**0**
King, broiled, 3 oz	114	17%	2	0	0
Pacific, broiled, 3 oz	171	45%	9	2	0
Spanish, broiled, 3 oz	134	36%	5	2	0
w/tomato sauce (Chicken of the Sea), ¼ cup	70	36%	3	1	2
MANGO, fresh, sliced, 1 cup	107	3%	0	0	25
MARGARINE & SPREADS					
Benecol, regular, 1 Tbs	70	100%	8	1	0
Benecol, light, 1 Tbs	50	100%	5	0.5	0
Blue Bonnet, regular stick, 1 Tbs	80	100%	9	3.5	0
Blue Bonnet, light stick, 1 Tbs	50	100%	5	1.5	0
Blue Bonnet, homestyle soft, 1 Tbs	60	100%	7	1	0
Blue Bonnet, homestyle, light, soft, 1 Tbs	40	100%	4.5	1	0
Country Crock, regular, tub & sticks, 1 Tbs	60	100%	7	2.5	0
Country Crock, churn style, 1 Tbs	80	100%	8	3	0
Country Crock, light, 1 Tbs	50	100%	5	1.5	0
Country Crock plus calcium, 1 Tbs	50	100%	5	1.5	0

Product and Portion Size	Calories	% Cal from Fat	Total Fat (g)	Bad Fat (g)	Net Carbs (g)
Fleischmann's, light, soft, 1 Tbs	40	100%	4.5	0	0
Fleischmann's, w/olive oil, soft tub, 1 Tbs	70	100%	8	1.5	0
Fleischmann's, original, soft, 1 Tbs	70	100%	8	1.5	0
I Can't Believe It's Not Butter, f-f, 1 Tbs	5	0%	0	0	0
I Can't Believe It's Not Butter, light, soft, 1 Tbs	50	100%	5	1	0
I Can't Believe It's Not Butter, orig., soft, 1 Tbs	80	100%	8	2	0
I Can't Believe It's Not Butter, spray, 5 sprays	0	0%	0	0	0
Parkay, light, tub, 1 Tbs	50	100%	5	1	0
Parkay, orig. stick, 1 Tbs	90	100%	10	4	0
Parkay orig. soft, tub, 1 Tbs	60	100%	7	1.5	0
Promise Buttery spread, soft, light, 1 Tbs	45	100%	5	1	0
Promise Buttery spread, soft, 1 Tbs	80	100%	8	1.5	0
Smart Balance, 67% light spread, 1 Tbs	80	100%	9	2.5	0
Smart Balance, 37% light spread, 1 Tbs	45	100%	5	1.5	0
Smart Balance Omega Plus, 1 Tbs	**80**	**100%**	**9**	**2.5**	**0**
MARSHMALLOWS					
Jet-puffed crème, ½ oz	45	0%	0	0	11
Jet-puffed, funmallows, 1 oz	100	0%	0	0	24

Product and Portion Size	Calories	% Cal from Fat	Total Fat (g)	Bad Fat (g)	Net Carbs (g)
Jet-pufffed, toasted coconut, 1 oz	100	25%	2.5	2	21
MAYONNAISE & SALAD DRESSING					
Hellman's canola, 1 Tbs	90	100%	10	1	0
Hellman's light, 1 Tbs	45	89%	4.5	0.5	0
Hellman's real mayonnaise, 1 Tbs	90	100%	10	1.5	0
Kraft f-f, 1 Tbs	10	0%	0	0	2
Kraft, light, 1 Tbs	40	88%	3.5	0.5	2
Kraft, real mayonnaise, 1 Tbs	100	100%	11	2	0
Miracle Whip, f-f, 1 Tbs	15	0%	0	0	3
Miracle Whip, light, 1 Tbs	25	60%	1.5	0	3
Miracle Whip dressing, 1 Tbs	40	75%	3.5	0.5	2
Smart Balance Omega Plus Light Mayo, 1 Tbs	**50**	**80%**	**5**	**0**	**2**
MILK					
1%, protein fortified, 1 cup	118	21%	3	2	14
2%, protein fortified, 1 cup	138	31%	5	3	14
Buttermilk, low-fat, 1 cup	98	19%	2	1	12
Chocolate, 2% (Organic Valley), 1 cup	170	26%	5	3	22
Evaporated nonfat, ½ cup	100	2%	0	0	15

Product and Portion Size	Calories	% Cal from Fat	Total Fat (g)	Bad Fat (g)	Net Carbs (g)
Evaporated, whole, ½ cup	169	50%	10	6	13
Hershey's 1% chocolate milk, 1 cup	120	13%	2.5	2	14
Lactose-free low-fat (Organic Valley), 1 cup	110	22%	2.5	1.5	14
Lactaid, f-f, 1 cup	80	0%	0	0	13
Lactaid, 2%, 1 cup	130	35%	5	3	12
Skim, calcium fortified, 1 cup	86	5%	0	0	12
Whole, 1 cup	146	48%	8	5	11
MIXED FRUIT					
Del Monte					
Cherry mixed, ½ cup	90	0%	0	0	21
Chunky mixed, ½ cup	100	0%	0	0	23
Fruit cocktail, ½ cup	100	0%	0	0	23
Fruit Naturals, tropical medley, ½ cup	70	0%	0	0	17
Lite chunky mixed, ½ cup	60	0%	0	0	14
Lite fruit cocktail, ½ cup	60	0%	0	0	14
Orchard Select, premium mixed, ½ cup	80	0%	0	0	19
Tropical fruit salad, ½ cup	60	0%	0	0	15
Dole					

Product and Portion Size	Calories	% Cal from Fat	Total Fat (g)	Bad Fat (g)	Net Carbs (g)
Mixed, frozen, ¾ cup	60	0%	0	0	14
Tropical mixed, ½ cup	90	0%	0	0	21
S&W					
Chunky mixed, natural style, ½ cup	80	0%	0	0	16
Cocktail, lite syrup, ½ cup	70	0%	0	0	17
Cocktail, natural style, ½ cup	80	0%	0	0	18
MOLASSES, blackstrap, 1 Tbs	47	0%	0	0	11
Regular, 1 Tbs	58	0%	0	0	7
MOUSSE					
Dr. Oetker, dark chocolate truffle, 2 Tbs mix	100	33%	3.5	3	14
Dr. Oetker, French vanilla, 2 Tbs mix	90	28%	3	2.5	15
Dr. Oetker, strawberry, 2 Tbs mix	80	31%	3	2.5	13
Nestle chocolate raspberry truffle, ¼ pkg	90	22%	2.5	1.5	12
Nestle dark chocolate, ¼ pkg	80	38%	3.5	2.5	11
Nestle milk chocolate, ¼ pkg	80	25%	2.5	2	15
MUFFINS (box/pouch mixes)					
Betty Crocker					
Apple streusel, ¼ cup mix	160	16%	3	1.5	33

Product and Portion Size	Calories	% Cal from Fat	Total Fat (g)	Bad Fat (g)	Net Carbs (g)
Authentic cornbread & muffin, 3 Tbs	110	5%	1	0	23
Banana nut, 3 Tbs mix	150	20%	3.5	1	26
Chocolate chip, pouch, ⅕ pouch	160	31%	5	3	25
Cinnamon streusel, 1/12 pkg	150	20%	3.5	2	28
Double chocolate, 1/12 pkg	190	32%	7	4	30
Lemon poppy seed, 1/12 pkg	140	14%	2	1	28
Lemon poppy seed, pouch, ⅙ pouch	130	23%	3.5	2	22
Triple berry, pouch, ⅙ pouch	120	21%	3	1.5	22
Twice the blueberries, ¼ cup mix	120	8%	1	0	25
Wild blueberry, 1/12 pkg	130	7%	1.5	0.5	26
Wild blueberry low fat, 3 Tbs	110	0%	0	0	26
Bob's Red Mill					
Date nut bran, 1 prep.	70	7%	0.5	0	11
Oat bran & date nut, 1 prep.	120	13%	1.5	0	20
Spice apple bran, 1 prep.	70	0%	0	0	13
Jiffy					
Apple cinnamon, ¼ cup mix	160	31%	6	2	25
Banana nut, ¼ cup mix	150	33%	6	2	23

Product and Portion Size	Calories	% Cal from Fat	Total Fat (g)	Bad Fat (g)	Net Carbs (g)
Blueberry, ¼ cup mix	170	29%	6	3	26
Bran, ¼ cup mix	140	29%	4.5	1.5	22
Raspberry, ¼ cup mix	170	29%	6	3	26
MUSHROOMS					
B in B canned, slices, 3 oz	30	33%	1.5	0.5	3
Brown or Italian, raw, 1 oz	6	0%	0	0	1
Green Giant, canned, whole or slices, ½ cup	25	0%	0	0	3
Portobello, raw, 1 cup diced	22	4%	0	0	3
Shiitake, cooked, no salt, 1 cup	81	4%	0	0	18
MUSSELS					
Blue, cooked, 3 oz	146	23%	4	1	6
Gold Seal, in cottonseed oil, whole, smoked, 2 oz	100	36%	4	1.5	2
MUSTARD					
Grey Poupon, country Dijon, 1 tsp	5	0%	0	0	0
Grey Poupon, honey mustard, 1 tsp	10	0%	0	0	2
Grey Poupon, spicy brown, 1 tsp	5	0%	0	0	0
Yellow, prepared, 1 tsp	3	39%	0	0	0
MUSTARD GREENS, cooked, 1 cup chopped	21	13%	0	0	0

Product and Portion Size	Calories	% Cal from Fat	Total Fat (g)	Bad Fat (g)	Net Carbs (g)
NECTARINE, 1 fruit 2.5" dia.	60	6%	0	0	12
NOODLES (dry)					
Light 'N Fluffy, macaroni dumpling, 2 oz	210	5%	1	0	40
Light 'N Fluffy, medium, 2 oz	210	12%	2.5	1	38
No Yolks, 2 oz	210	2%	0.5	0	38
Pennsylvania Dutch, medium egg, 1 cup	220	14%	3	1	38
NOODLE DISHES (box mix); also see Pasta					
Lipton Asian Sides, Teriyaki, ⅔ cup mix	240	8%	2	0	47
Lipton Pasta Sides, alfredo, ⅔ cup mix	240	17%	4.5	2.5	39
Lipton Pasta Sides, beef, ⅔ cup mix	210	5%	1	0	42
Lipton Pasta Sides, butter, ⅔ cup mix	240	15%	4	2	47
Lipton Pasta Sides, cheddar broccoli, mix	250	10%	3	1	45
Lipton Pasta Sides, chicken, ⅔ cup mix	220	9%	2	0	42
Lipton Pasta Sides, stroganoff, mix	210	9%	2	1	38
OCEAN PERCH, Atlantic, broiled, 3 oz	103	16%	2	0	0
OILS					
Avocado, corn, **sesame, soybean,** 1 Tbs	**120**	**100%**	**14**	**2**	**0**
Almond, **canola,** sunflower, **walnut,** 1 Tbs	**120**	**100%**	**14**	**1**	**0**

Product and Portion Size	Calories	% Cal from Fat	Total Fat (g)	Bad Fat (g)	Net Carbs (g)
Mazola Right Blend (corn & canola), 1 Tbs	120	100%	14	1	0
OKRA, cooked, no salt, ½ cup slices	18	6%	0	0	2
OLIVES					
Lindsay, black, large, 4	**25**	**80%**	**2.5**	**0**	**1**
Lindsay, green, medium, 5	**25**	**80%**	**2.5**	**0**	**1**
Lindsay, green, slices w/pimentos, 2 Tbs	**25**	**80%**	**2.5**	**0**	**<1**
Lindsay, kalamata, 3	**25**	**80%**	**2.5**	**0**	**<1**
ONIONS					
Fresh, chopped, yellow or red, 1 cup	67	2%	0	0	14
Fresh, tops and bulbs (scallions), 1 cup	32	5%	0	0	4
Ore-Ida, frozen, Gourmet rings, 3 pcs	180	39%	8	1	24
Ore-Ida, frozen, Vidalia Os, 4 pcs	180	50%	10	1.5	21
ORANGES					
Fresh, California, 2⅝" dia.	59	5%	0	0	11
Fresh, Florida, 2⅝" dia.	65	4%	0	0	13
Mandarin, canned (Dole), ½ cup	80	0%	0	0	18
ORANGE JUICE/BEVERAGE					
Cascadian Farm, frozen, organic, 8 oz prep.	110	0%	0	0	27

Product and Portion Size	Calories	% Cal from Fat	Total Fat (g)	Bad Fat (g)	Net Carbs (g)
Dole, 100%, 8 oz	120	0%	0	0	27
Dole, orange, peach, mango, 8 oz	120	0%	0	0	28
Minute Maid, country style, 8 oz	110	0%	0	0	27
Minute Maid, home style & calcium & vit. D, 8 oz	110	0%	0	0	27
Minute Maid, orange passion, 8 oz	130	0%	0	0	31
Minute Maid, orange tangerine, 8 oz	110	0%	0	0	27
Tang, orange, 8 oz prep.	90	0%	0	0	23
Tang, orange pineapple, 8 oz prep.	100	0%	0	0	24
Tang, orange, sugar free, 8 oz prep.	5	0%	0	0	0
Tropicana, calcium & vit. D, 8 oz	110	0%	0	0	26
Tropicana, Essentials Light 'N Healthy, 8 oz	50	0%	0	0	13
Tropicana, Essentials Fiber, 8 oz	120	0%	0	0	29
Tropicana, original, 8 oz	110	0%	0	0	26
OYSTERS					
Canned, smoked, in oil, 3.75 oz can	140	50%	8	2	8
Canned, whole, 2 oz	80	38%	3	1	6
Eastern, raw, 1 cup	169	33%	6	2	10
Pacific, raw, 3 oz	69	26%	2	0	4

Product and Portion Size	Calories	% Cal from Fat	Total Fat (g)	Bad Fat (g)	Net Carbs (g)
PANCAKE/WAFFLE (mix)					
Aunt Jemima, buckwheat, ¼ cup mix	100	10%	1	0	20
Aunt Jemima, buttermilk complete, ⅓ cup mix	160	13%	2	0.5	30
Aunt Jemima, original, ⅓ cup mix	150	3%	0.5	0	32
Aunt Jemima, original complete, ⅓ cup mix	160	9%	1.5	0	31
Aunt Jemima, whole wheat, ¼ cup mix	120	4%	0.5	0	23
Bisquick Shake 'n Pour buttermilk mix, ½ cup	200	12%	3	1	38
Hungry Jack, buttermilk, ⅓ cup mix	150	10%	1.5	0	30
Hungry Jack, extra light & fluffy, ⅓ cup mix	150	13%	2	0	29
Hungry Jack, original, ⅓ cup mix	150	10%	1.5	0	30
Krusteaz, blueberry, ½ cup mix	240	10%	2.5	1	45
Krusteaz, buttermilk, ½ cup mix	210	10%	2	0.5	41
PANCAKE/WAFFLE (frozen)					
Aunt Jemima, homestyle waffles, 2	190	24%	5	1	31
Aunt Jemima magic mini pancakes, cinnamon, 13	240	15%	4	1	44
Aunt Jemima magic mini pancakes, strawberry, 13	240	15%	4	1	44
Eggo, apple cinnamon, blueberry, or strawberry waffles, 2	190	26%	6	1.5	29
Eggo, buttermilk pancakes, 3	280	29%	9	1.5	43

Product and Portion Size	Calories	% Cal from Fat	Total Fat (g)	Bad Fat (g)	Net Carbs (g)
Eggo, buttermilk waffles, 2	180	28%	6	3.5	25
Eggo, chocolate chip waffles, 2	200	25%	6	3.5	31
Eggo, Choco-'Nilla Flip-Flop waffles, 2	190	32%	7	4	27
Eggo, Special K waffles, 2	190	53%	11	4	8
Pillsbury					
Blueberry pancakes, 3	240	15%	4	2	44
Buttermilk pancakes, 3	240	17%	4	2	45
Chocolate chip pancakes, 3	270	19%	5	3	48
Mini blueberry pancakes w/syrup, 14 cakes	420	14%	7	3	85
Mini buttermilk pancakes, w/syrup, 14 cakes	410	15%	7	3	83
Original pancakes, 3	240	15%	4	2	45
Waffles, blueberry, 2	190	24%	5	3	31
Waffles, buttermilk, 2	170	26%	5	3	27
Waffles, homestyle, 2	170	26%	5	3	28
Waffle sticks, blueberry w/syrup, 6	340	18%	7	3.5	66
Waffle sticks, chocolate chip w/syrup, 6	350	17%	7	3.5	67
Waffle sticks, cinnamon w/syrup, 6	330	18%	6	3.5	63
PANCAKE SYRUP					
Aunt Jemima, butter lite, ¼ cup	100	0%	0	0	26

Product and Portion Size	Calories	% Cal from Fat	Total Fat (g)	Bad Fat (g)	Net Carbs (g)
Aunt Jemima, butter rich, ¼ cup	210	0%	0	0	53
Aunt Jemima, lite, ¼ cup	100	0%	0	0	26
Aunt Jemima, original, ¼ cup	210	0%	0	0	52
Log Cabin, sugar free, ¼ cup	35	0%	0	0	12
Maple Grove Farms, ¼ cup	200	0%	0	0	53
Vermont Maid, ¼ cup	210	0%	0	0	53
PALM, hearts, canned (Haddon House), 1.5 sticks	20	0%	0	0	1
PAPAYA					
Fresh, cubed, 1 cup	55	3%	0	0	11
Nectar (Knudsen), 8 oz	140	0%	0	0	35
Nectar, creamed, 8 oz	40	0%	0	0	8
PARSNIPS, fresh, cooked, no salt, ½ cup	55	4%	0	0	10
PASTA—Bowls/Boxes					
Betty Crocker					
Bowl Appetit, cheddar, broccoli, pasta, 1 bowl	330	27%	11	6.5	47
Bowl Appetit, chicken pasta, 1 bowl	260	23%	6	3	40
Bowl Appetit, garlic parmesan pasta, 1 bowl	320	25%	9	5.5	49
Bowl Appetit, pasta alfredo, 1 bowl	360	28%	11	7.5	52
Bowl Appetit, three-cheese rotini, 1 bowl	360	25%	10	6.5	53

Product and Portion Size	Calories	% Cal from Fat	Total Fat (g)	Bad Fat (g)	Net Carbs (g)
Chicken Helper, cheddar & broccoli, ½ cup mix	160	25%	4.5	3	23
Chicken Helper, chicken fettuccine, ½ cup mix	140	18%	3	2	24
Chicken Helper, four cheese, ⅔ cup mix	160	28%	5	3.5	23
Cookbook Favorite chicken fettuccini, ⅓ cup mix	180	28%	6	2	24
Cookbook Favorite garlic & herb chicken penne, ⅓ cup mix	150	33%	5	1	19
Suddenly Pasta Salad, Caesar, ½ cup pkg	170	6%	1	0	33
Suddenly Pasta Salad, classic, ⅔ cup pkg	180	6%	1	0	35
Suddenly Pasta Salad, creamy Italian, ⅓ cup pkg	160	6%	1.5	0	30
Suddenly Pasta Salad, ranch & bacon, ½ cup pkg	160	6%	1.5	0	30
Tuna Helper, cheesy pasta, ¾ cup mix	150	10%	1.5	1	29
Tuna Helper, creamy broccoli, ½ cup mix	190	24%	5	1.5	30
Tuna Helper, creamy parmesan, ¾ cup mix	180	14%	2.5	1.5	31
Tuna Helper, creamy pasta, ¾ cup mix	180	28%	5	3.5	29
Tuna Helper, fettucini alfredo, ¾ cup mix	170	18%	3	2	29
Canned					
Campbell's beef ravioli in meat sauce, 1 cup	270	27%	8	3.5	34
Campbell's spaghetti in tomato & cheese, 1 cup	200	7%	1.5	0.5	37

Product and Portion Size	Calories	% Cal from Fat	Total Fat (g)	Bad Fat (g)	Net Carbs (g)
Chef Boyardee ABS, 123s w/meatballs, 1 cup	270	33%	10	4.5	32
Chef Boyardee mini beef ravioli, meat sauce, 1 cup	240	29%	8	3.5	30
Chef Boyardee mini shells w/meatballs, 1 cup	260	35%	10	4.5	30
Chef Boyardee mini spaghetti w/meatballs, 1 cup	270	33%	10	4.5	30
SpaghettiOs, 1 cup	180	5%	1	0.5	34
SpaghettiOs, A to Z w/meatballs, 1 cup	260	31%	9	3.5	30
SpaghettiOs, A to Z, w/sliced franks, 1 cup	230	27%	7	2.5	31
SpaghettiOs, w/meatballs, 1 cup	240	30%	8	3.5	29
SpaghettiOs plus calcium, 1 cup	170	5%	1	0.5	32
Dry					
Corn, angel hair (Westbrae), 2 oz	210	7%	1.5	0	46
Durum wheat, various brands, 2 oz	210	4%	1	0	40
Kamut, organic (Eden Foods), 2 oz	210	7%	1.5	0.5	32
Rye, organic (Eden Foods), 2 oz	200	0%	0	0	36
Spinach spaghetti (Westbrae), 2 oz	180	11%	2	0	30
Whole wheat (DeCecco), 2 oz	180	8%	1.5	0	28
Whole-wheat lasagna (Westbrae), 2 oz	180	6%	1.5	0	27
Whole-wheat spaghetti (Westbrae), 2 oz	200	7%	1.5	0	30

Product and Portion Size	Calories	% Cal from Fat	Total Fat (g)	Bad Fat (g)	Net Carbs (g)
Refrigerated—Buitoni					
Angel hair pasta, 1 cup	230	11%	2.5	1	41
Linguine, 1¼ cup	240	10%	2.5	1	43
Ravioli, classic beef, 1¼ cup	350	29%	11	3.5	45
Ravioli, four cheese, 1⅓ cup	330	27%	10	6	42
Ravioli, garden vegetable, 1 cup	250	18%	5	2	38
Tortellini, cheese & roasted garlic, 1 cup	270	26%	8	4	36
Tortellini, mozzarella & pepperoni, 1 cup	330	27%	10	4.5	42
Tortellini, spinach cheese, 1 cup	320	19%	7	3.5	46
Tortellini, sweet Italian sausage, 1 cup	330	27%	10	3	45
Tortellini, three cheese, 1 cup	330	21%	8	3.5	47
PASTA SAUCE					
Buitoni					
Alfredo, ½ cup	140	71%	11	7	5
Light, ½ cup	80	56%	5	3.5	5
Marinara, ½ cup	70	36%	3	0.5	8
Pesto w/basil, ¼ cup	300	83%	28	5	4
Tomato herb parmesan, ½ cup	130	54%	8	2.5	8

Product and Portion Size	Calories	% Cal from Fat	Total Fat (g)	Bad Fat (g)	Net Carbs (g)
Classico					
Alfredo, ¼ cup	120	83%	11	5	3
Basil pesto, ¼ cup	230	83%	21	3	5
Florentine spinach & cheese, ½ cup	80	56%	5	1	4
Italian sausage w/pepper & onion, ½ cup	90	22%	2	1	11
Roasted garlic, ½ cup	60	17%	1	0	9
Tomato & basil, ½ cup	60	17%	1	0	9
Del Monte					
Italian herb chunky, ½ cup	60	17%	1	0	11
Spaghetti sauce w/four cheeses, ½ cup	70	14%	1.5	0	12
Spaghetti sauce w/meat, ½ cup	60	17%	1	0	11
Spaghetti sauce w/mushrooms, ½ cup	60	8%	0.5	0	12
DiGiorno Microwaveable					
Alfredo, 2.5 oz	180	89%	17	3	3
Alfredo, four cheese, 2.5 oz	160	81%	15	6	3
Alfredo, reduced fat, 2.5 oz	130	54%	8	5	10
Basil pesto, 2.3 oz	310	90%	31	5	5
Marinara, 3.5 oz	70	21%	1.5	0	10

Product and Portion Size	Calories	% Cal from Fat	Total Fat (g)	Bad Fat (g)	Net Carbs (g)
Eden Foods					
Pizza pasta sauce, organic, ½ cup	65	38%	2.5	0	4
Spaghetti sauce, organic, ½ cup	80	25%	2.5	0	9
Hunt's					
Four cheese, ½ cup	50	20%	1	0	7
Meat, ½ cup	60	17%	1	0	8
Mushroom, ½ cup	45	11%	0.5	0	7
Muir Glen Organic					
Fire roasted tomato, ½ cup	70	21%	2	0	9
Four cheese, ½ cup	80	25%	3	1	9
Garden vegetable, ½ cup	60	8%	1	0	8
Mushroom marinara, ½ cup	50	0%	0	0	8
Tomato basil, ½ cup	60	8%	1	0	10
Newman's Own					
Bombolina, ½ cup	90	44%	4.5	0.5	12
Five cheese, ½ cup	80	38%	3	1.5	9
Italian sausage & pepper, ½ cup	90	39%	4	1	10
Marinara, ½ cup	70	29%	2	0	11

Product and Portion Size	Calories	% Cal from Fat	Total Fat (g)	Bad Fat (g)	Net Carbs (g)
Pesto & tomato, ½ cup	80	44%	4	0.5	9
Vodka sauce, ½ cup	110	41%	5	1.5	11
Prego					
Chunky garden, mushroom supreme, ½ cup	120	30%	4	1	15
Chunky garden, tomato, onion & garlic, ½ cup	110	28%	3.5	0.5	13
Fresh mushroom, ½ cup	120	26%	3.5	1	15
Hearty meat, three meat supreme, ½ cup	170	53%	10	4	10
Italian sausage & garlic, ½ cup	120	38%	5	1.5	13
Organic mushroom, ½ cup	90	24%	2.5	0	9
Roasted garlic parmesan, ½ cup	100	9%	1	0.5	13
Progresso					
Lobster, ½ cup	100	60%	7	1	4
Red clam, ½ cup	60	17%	1	0	7
White clam, ½ cup	130	68%	10	1.5	5
Ragu					
Chunky, sundried tomato & basil, ½ cup	120	21%	3	0	19
Chunky super vegetable primavera, ½ cup	110	23%	3	0	15
Light, tomato & basil, ½ cup	60	0%	0	0	10

Product and Portion Size	Calories	% Cal from Fat	Total Fat (g)	Bad Fat (g)	Net Carbs (g)
Organic cheese, ½ cup	80	31%	3	0.5	9
Robusto, parmesan & romano, ½ cup	90	28%	3	0.5	10
PASTRAMI					
Beef, 98% f-f, 2 oz	54	11%	1	0	1
Carl Buddig, beef, chopped, pressed, 2 oz	80	41%	4	2	1
Sara Lee beef, pre-sliced, 2 slices	60	33%	2.5	1	0
PASTRY—Toaster					
Kellogg's Pop Tarts					
Apple cinnamon, 1	210	24%	6	3	36
Blueberry, 1	210	24%	6	3	36
Chocolate chip cookie dough, 1	200	23%	5	2.5	34
French toast, 1	220	32%	8	4	34
Frosted cherry, 1	200	23%	5	2.5	37
Frosted chocolate fudge, 1	200	23%	5	2.5	36
Frosted cookies & crème, 1	200	23%	5	2.5	36
Frosted raspberry, 1	210	21%	5	2.5	37
Frosted S'mores, 1	200	23%	5	2.5	35
Low-fat frosted brown sugar cinnamon, 1	190	13%	3	1.5	37

Product and Portion Size	Calories	% Cal from Fat	Total Fat (g)	Bad Fat (g)	Net Carbs (g)
Low-fat frosted chocolate fudge, 1	190	13%	3	1.5	37
Pillsbury Toaster Strudel					
Apple, 1	190	42%	9	4.5	24
Blueberry, 1	190	42%	9	4.5	25
Brown sugar cinnamon, 1	200	40%	9	4.5	27
Chocolate fudge, 1	210	43%	10	5.5	25
Cream cheese, 1	200	50%	11	6	23
Cream cheese & raspberry, 1	200	45%	10	5	24
S'Mores, 1	200	40%	9	4.5	26
Strawberry, 1	190	42%	9	4.5	24
Wild berry, 1	190	42%	9	4.5	24
PEACHES, fresh, raw, 1 2.5" dia.	38	5%	0	0	8
Canned					
Del Monte, carb clever, sliced, ½ cup	30	0%	0	0	6
Del Monte, freestone slices, ½ cup	100	0%	0	0	23
Del Monte fruit naturals, chunks, ½ cup	70	0%	0	0	16
Del Monte harvest spice, sliced, ½ cup	80	0%	0	0	20
S&W, halves, ½ cup	70	0%	0	0	16

Product and Portion Size	Calories	% Cal from Fat	Total Fat (g)	Bad Fat (g)	Net Carbs (g)
S&W, natural style, ½ cup	80	0%	0	0	18
S&W snow beaches, ½ cup	80	0%	0	0	19
Dried, sulfured, halves, 1 cup	382	3%	2	0	85
Frozen, Cascadian Farm, sliced, organic, 1 cup	60	0%	0	0	13
Juice/nectar					
Knudsen, 8 oz	130	0%	0	0	31
Santa Cruz, organic, 8 oz	120	0%	0	0	29
PEANUT BUTTER					
Jif, creamy, 2 Tbs	**190**	**68%**	**16**	**3**	**5**
Jif, creamy & honey, 2 Tbs	**190**	**68%**	**15**	**2.5**	**9**
Jif, reduced fat, 2 Tbs	**190**	**58%**	**12**	**2.5**	**13**
Maranatha organic, creamy, 2 Tbs	**190**	**79%**	**16**	**2.5**	**5**
Maranatha organic, crunchy, 2 Tbs	**190**	**79%**	**16**	**2.5**	**5**
Peter Pan, creamy, 2 Tbs	**190**	**74%**	**17**	**3.5**	**4**
Skippy, honey roasted creamy, 2 Tbs	**190**	**74%**	**17**	**3.5**	**5**
Skippy, reduced fat, creamy, 2 Tbs	**190**	**52%**	**12**	**2.5**	**13**
Skippy, regular creamy, 2 Tbs	**190**	**74%**	**16**	**3**	**5**
Skippy, super chunk, 2 Tbs	**190**	**79%**	**17**	**3.5**	**5**
Smart Balance omega, creamy, 2 Tbs	**190**	**74%**	**16**	**2.5**	**4**

Product and Portion Size	Calories	% Cal from Fat	Total Fat (g)	Bad Fat (g)	Net Carbs (g)
Smucker's natural, creamy or chunky, 2 Tbs	**210**	**71%**	**16**	**2.5**	**4**
Smucker's natural, reduced fat creamy, 2 Tbs	**200**	**55%**	**12**	**2**	**10**
PEANUTS					
Dry roasted, w/salt, 1 oz	**165**	**71%**	**14**	**2**	**4**
Oil roasted, w/salt, 1 oz	**169**	**73%**	**15**	**2**	**1**
Planters, honey roasted, 1 oz	**160**	**69%**	**13**	**1.5**	**6**
Planters, sweet 'n crunchy, 1 oz	**140**	**43%**	**7**	**1**	**14**
PEARS, fresh, raw, 1 medium	96	2%	0	0	21
Canned/jarred					
Del Monte, bartlett, cinnamon halves, ½ cup	80	0%	0	0	20
Del Monte, bartlett, halves, light syrup, ½ cup	60	0%	0	0	14
Del Monte, bartlett, Orchard Select, ½ cup	80	0%	0	0	18
S&W, bartlett, halves, light syrup, ½ cup	80	0%	0	0	17
S&W, bartlett, slices, natural style, ½ cup	80	0%	0	0	19
Nectar, Santa Cruz, organic, 8 oz	120	0%	0	0	30
PEAS, fresh, boiled, no salt, 1 cup	134	2%	0	0	16
Canned					
Del Monte, peas & carrots, ½ cup	60	0%	0	0	9
Del Monte, sweet peas, ½ cup	60	0%	0	0	9

Product and Portion Size	Calories	% Cal from Fat	Total Fat (g)	Bad Fat (g)	Net Carbs (g)
Del Monte, very young small sweet, ½ cup	60	0%	0	0	6
Green Giant, LeSueur early peas, ⅔ cup	60	8%	0.5	0	7
Stokely, peas & pearl onions, ½ cup	40	0%	0	0	7
Frozen					
Green Giant, baby sweet peas & butter, ¾ cup	90	17%	1.5	0.5	10
Green Giant, select early June peas, ⅔ cup	60	8%	0.5	0	7
Green Giant, sugar snap peas, ½ cup	40	0%	0	0	8
Green Giant, sweet w/tiny pearl onions, ½ cup	60	0%	0	0	8
PECANS					
Planters, chips, 2 oz	**390**	**92%**	**40**	**3**	**2**
Planters, fresh, unsalted halves, 1 oz	**190**	**89%**	**20**	**1.5**	**1**
PEPPERS					
Bruno, banana wax pepper, 4 pcs	10	0%	0	0	1
Bruno, mild wax peppers, 11 pcs	8	0%	0	0	1
Fresh, raw, green, chopped, 1 cup	30	7%	0	0	4
Fresh, raw, red, chopped, 1 cup	39	10%	0	0	6
Fresh, raw, yellow, large, 3" dia.	50	7%	0	0	10
Vlasic, pepper rings, 12	5	0%	0	0	1

Product and Portion Size	Calories	% Cal from Fat	Total Fat (g)	Bad Fat (g)	Net Carbs (g)
Vlasic, zesty cherry peppers, 2	10	0%	0	0	2
PEPPERONI					
Hormel, original 14 slices	140	86%	13	6	0
Smart Deli, slices (soy), 13 slices	45	0%	0	0	2
PICKLES					
Cascadian Farms, baby dills, 1⅓ pickle	5	0%	0	0	1
Cascadian Farms, bread & butter chips, 5 slices	30	0%	0	0	8
Claussen bread 'n butter, sandwich slices, 1 oz	5	0%	0	0	5
Claussen half sours, NY deli style, 1 oz	5	0%	0	0	1
Claussen kosher dill halves, 1 oz	5	0%	0	0	1
Claussen kosher dill spears, 1 oz	5	0%	0	0	1
Claussen kosher dill burger slices, 1 oz	5	0%	0	0	1
Claussen sweet gerkins, 1 oz	30	0%	0	0	7
Del Monte, sweet, midget, 1 oz	40	0%	0	0	9
Del Monte, sweet, whole, 1 oz	40	0%	0	0	9
PIES—Frozen					
Edward's chocolate butter pecan, 1 pc	560	43%	32	14	61
Edward's chocolate cream, ⅛ pie	450	53%	27	18.5	47

Product and Portion Size	Calories	% Cal from Fat	Total Fat (g)	Bad Fat (g)	Net Carbs (g)
Edward's Georgia pecan, ⅛ pie	490	49%	26	8	59
Edward's key lime, ⅛ pie	450	42%	22	16.5	58
Edward's Oreo cream, ⅛ pie	480	56%	30	20.5	49
Edward's turtle, ⅛ pie	390	51%	22	13.5	45
Marie Callender, apple, 1/10 pie	350	49%	19	9.5	41
Marie Callender, pumpkin, ⅛ pie	330	36%	14	6	44
Mrs. Smith, blueberry, ⅛ pie	330	45%	16	7	42
Mrs. Smith, cherry, ⅛ pie	330	45%	16	7	43
Mrs. Smith, coconut custard, ⅛ pie	290	48%	16	8.5	30
Mrs. Smith, sweet potato, ⅛ pie	350	46%	18	7	43
Sara Lee, apple, ⅛ pie	340	41%	15	7	49
Sara Lee, blueberry, ⅛ pie	350	40%	15	7	49
Sara Lee, Dutch apple, ⅛ pie	340	38%	14	6	50
PIE CRUST					
Pet-Ritz, deep dish, ⅛ crust	90	50%	5	2	11
Pet-Ritz, deep dish, all vegetable, ⅛ crust	90	50%	5	2.5	11
Pet-Ritz, regular, ⅛ crust	80	44%	4	1.5	9
Pillsbury all ready rolled, ⅛ crust	120	50%	7	2.5	13

Product and Portion Size	Calories	% Cal from Fat	Total Fat (g)	Bad Fat (g)	Net Carbs (g)
PIE FILLING					
Comstock					
Apple, ½ cup	30	0%	0	0	5
Blueberry, more fruit, ½ cup	100	0%	0	0	22
Cherry, more fruit, ½ cup	100	0%	0	0	22
Lucky Leaf					
Apple, ⅓ cup	90	0%	0	0	20
Apricot, ⅓ cup	90	0%	0	0	22
Blueberry, premium, ⅓ cup	100	0%	0	0	23
Coconut crème, ⅓ cup	100	10%	2	0	22
Lemon cream, ⅓ cup	130	8%	1	0	31
Pineapple, ⅓ cup	100	0%	0	0	22
Raisin, ⅓ cup	90	0%	0	0	22
Strawberry, premium, ½ cup	100	0%	0	0	22
PIEROGIES					
Mrs. T, American cheese, 3	210	24%	6	3	31
Mrs. T, broccoli & cheddar, 3	200	20%	4.5	2	31
Mrs. T, four cheese, 3	230	26%	7	1.5	35

Product and Portion Size	Calories	% Cal from Fat	Total Fat (g)	Bad Fat (g)	Net Carbs (g)
Mrs. T, sour cream, 3	210	24%	6	3	31
PINEAPPLE, fresh, diced, 1 cup	74	2%	0	0	18
Del Monte, chunks in heavy syrup, ½ cup	90	0%	0	0	23
Del Monte, chunks in own juice, ½ cup	70	0%	0	0	16
Del Monte, crushed, heavy syrup, ½ cup	90	0%	0	0	23
Del Monte, Fruit Naturals, ½ cup	70	0%	0	0	17
Dole, fruit bowl, 4 oz	60	0%	0	0	15
Dole, fruit bowl in lime gel, 4.3 oz	90	0%	0	0	23
Dole, slices in 100% juice, 2 slices	60	0%	0	0	14
Dole, tidbits in 100% juice, ½ cup	60	0%	0	0	14
PINEAPPLE JUICE/BEVERAGE					
Dole 100%, 8 oz	120	0%	0	0	29
Dole, pineapple orange, 100%, 6 oz	100	0%	0	0	24
Knudsen, nectar, 8 oz	140	0%	0	0	46
Knudsen, pineapple coconut, 8 oz	130	4%	1	0.5	31
Santa Cruz, orange pineapple, 8 oz	130	0%	0	0	31
Santa Cruz, pineapple coconut, 8 oz	130	4%	1.0	1	30
PISTACHIOS, dry roasted (Planters), 1 oz	**170**	**76%**	**14**	**2**	**3**

Product and Portion Size	Calories	% Cal from Fat	Total Fat (g)	Bad Fat (g)	Net Carbs (g)
PIZZA (frozen); also see FAST FOOD					
Amy's Kitchen					
Cheese, ⅓ pie	310	35%	12	4	36
Mediterranean w/cornmeal crust, ⅓ pie	360	39%	15	4.5	42
Pesto, ⅓ pie	310	35%	12	3.5	37
Rice crust, cheese, ⅓ pie	300	43%	14	4	29
Roasted vegetable, ⅓ pie	270	30%	9	1.5	40
Soy cheese, ⅓ pie	290	34%	11	1	35
Three cheese w/cornmeal crust, ⅓ pie	370	46%	19	4	39
DiGiorno					
Cheese stuffed crust, ⅙ pie	350	43%	16	7	32
Cheese stuffed crust, 3 meat, ⅙ pie	340	41%	16	7.5	32
Cheese stuffed crust, pepperoni, ⅕ pie	370	38%	16	8.5	37
Cheese stuffed crust, 4 cheese, ⅕ pie	360	36%	14	8.5	38
Deep dish, 3 meat, ⅙ pie	310	42%	15	7.5	30
Deep dish, pepperoni, ⅙ pie	340	47%	18	8.5	30
Deep dish, supreme, ⅙ pie	320	44%	15	7.5	31
Microwave rising crust, pepperoni, ½ pie	390	41%	18	8.5	41

Product and Portion Size	Calories	% Cal from Fat	Total Fat (g)	Bad Fat (g)	Net Carbs (g)
Microwave rising crust, supreme, ½ pie	400	40%	18	8.5	41
Thin crispy crust, 4 meat, ⅕ pie	320	38%	13	5	35
Thin crispy crust, harvest wheat supreme, ⅕ pie	250	28%	8	3.5	28
Thin crispy crust, harvest wheat pepperoni, ⅕ pie	270	30%	9	4	28
Thin crispy crust, supreme, ⅕ pie	300	33%	12	5	33
Jeno's Crisp'n Tasty					
Canadian bacon, 1 pizza	420	38%	18	8	47
Cheese, 1 pizza	440	43%	21	10	45
Combination, 1 pizza	490	47%	25	10.5	48
Hamburger, 1 pizza	480	42%	22	9.5	48
Pepperoni, 1 pizza	490	47%	26	11	48
Sausage, 1 pizza	480	46%	24	10.5	48
Supreme, 1 pizza	490	47%	25	10.5	47
Three meat, 1 pizza	480	44%	24	10.5	47
Lean Cuisine					
Cheese French bread, 1 pkg	320	19%	7	4	44
Delux French bread, 1 pkg	310	26%	9	3.5	41
Pepperoni French bread, 1 pkg	300	20%	7	2.5	42

Product and Portion Size	Calories	% Cal from Fat	Total Fat (g)	Bad Fat (g)	Net Carbs (g)
Tombstone					
Brickoven pepperoni, ¼ pizza	310	45%	16	7	27
Brickoven pepperoni & sausage, ¼ pizza	320	47%	16	7	27
Brickoven, supreme, ¼ pizza	320	44%	16	7	27
Double top pepperoni, ⅕ pizza	400	50%	22	10.5	27
Harvest wheat thin crust, cheese, ⅓ pizza	300	30%	10	5	33
Harvest wheat thin crust, supreme, ¼ pizza	260	35%	10	4.5	26
Light veggie, ⅕ pizza	230	22%	6	2	27
Original, extra cheese, ¼ pizza	350	40%	15	8.5	33
Original, sausage, ⅕ pizza	290	38%	13	5	27
Original, supreme, ⅕ pizza	300	40%	14	6	28
Original, 4 meat, ⅕ pizza	310	42%	14	6	27
Totino's Party Pizza					
Canadian bacon, ½ pizza	320	41%	15	7	33
Cheese, ½ pizza	320	44%	15	7	33
Combination, ½ pizza	380	50%	21	9	33
Hamburger, ½ pizza	360	47%	19	9	34
Mexican, ½ pizza	370	46%	19	9	32

Product and Portion Size	Calories	% Cal from Fat	Total Fat (g)	Bad Fat (g)	Net Carbs (g)
Mini meatball, ½ pizza	350	46%	18	8	33
Pepperoni, ½ pizza	360	50%	20	9	30
Sausage, ½ pizza	360	47%	19	8	33
Supreme, ½ pizza	360	47%	19	8.5	33
Three cheese, ½ pizza	330	42%	16	7.5	32
Three meat, ½ pizza	350	46%	18	8	33
PIZZA SNACKS					
Totino's Mexican style, chicken fajita, 6 rolls	190	26%	6	3	24
Totino's Mexican style, chicken & cheese, 6 rolls	190	26%	7	3	23
Totino's pizza rolls, cheese, 6 rolls	190	26%	6	3	25
Totino's pizza rolls, cheesy taco, 6 rolls	210	43%	10	5	22
Totino's pizza rolls, combination, 6 rolls	220	45%	11	4.5	23
Totino's pizza rolls, pepperoni, 6 rolls	210	43%	10	4	24
Totino's pizza rolls, sausage, 6 rolls	210	43%	10	4	23
Totino's pizza rolls, supreme, 6 rolls	210	38%	9	3.5	23
Totino's pizza rolls, three meat, 6 rolls	210	38%	9	4	23
PLANTAIN, raw, 1 cup	181	3%	1	0	44
PLUMS, raw, one 2⅛" dia.	30	5%	0	0	7
Canned, purple, light syrup, 1 cup	159	1%	0	0	39

Product and Portion Size	Calories	% Cal from Fat	Total Fat (g)	Bad Fat (g)	Net Carbs (g)
POMEGRANATE					
Fresh, ½ fruit	80	5%	0.5	0	17
Knudsen, Just pomegranate, 8 oz	150	0%	0	0	38
Knudsen, Vita pomegranate, 8 oz	130	0%	0	0	33
POM, 100%, 8 oz	160	0%	0	0	40
POPCORN					
Air-popped, plain, no salt, 1 cup	31	9%	0	0	5
Healthy Choice, microwave, butter, 3 Tbs kernels	120	20%	3	0	20
Healthy Choice, microwave, natural, 3 Tbs kernels	120	20%	2.5	0	21
Jolly Time, microwave, healthy pop, 2 Tbs kernel	90	22%	2	0	14
Jolly Time, microwave, sassy salsa, 2 Tbs kernels	180	67%	13	9	12
Jolly Time, microwave, mallow magic, 2 Tbs kernels	180	67%	13	2.5	12
Orville Redenbacher, butter, 3 Tbs kernels	170	65%	12	6	14
Orville Redenbacher, movie theater, 3 Tbs kernels	170	65%	12	6	13
Orville Redenbacher, smart pop, 3 Tbs kernels	130	15%	2.5	0.5	23
Orville Redenbacher, tender white, 3 Tbs kernels	180	67%	13	7	12
Wise, bagged, butter flavored, 1 oz	150	60%	10	2	11
Wise, bagged, hot cheese, 1 oz	150	60%	10	2	12
Wise, bagged, lite butter flavored, 1 oz	140	32%	5	2.5	19

Product and Portion Size	Calories	% Cal from Fat	Total Fat (g)	Bad Fat (g)	Net Carbs (g)
PORK					
Fresh, center loin chops, lean & fat, broiled, 3 oz	204	49%	11	4	0
Fresh, center rib chops, lean & fat, broiled, 3 oz	224	53%	13	5	0
Fresh, center rib roast, lean, roasted, 3 oz	182	43%	9	3	0
Fresh, loin blade chops, lean & fat, broiled, 3 oz	272	70%	21	8	0
Fresh, spare ribs, braised, lean & fat, 3 oz	337	69%	26	9	0
Fresh, tenderloin, lean, roasted, 3 oz	139	26%	4	1	0
Fresh, tenderloin, lean & fat, roasted, 3 oz	147	32%	5	2	0
Hormel Always Tender, boneless loin, 4 oz	162	45%	8	3	1
Hormel Always Tender, center chops, 4 oz	187	52%	11	4	1
PORK RINDS					
Wise, hot & spicy, BBQ, 0.625 oz	90	50%	5	1.5	1
Wise, original, 0.625 oz	90	56%	6	2	0
Wise, sweet & mild BBQ, 0.625 oz	90	56%	6	2	1
POTATOES (white)					
Baked, skin & flesh, 1 medium 2¼–3¼ dia.	161	1%	0	0	33
Boiled, skin & flesh, 2½ dia.	118	1%	0	0	25
Canned					
Del Monte, au gratin, ½ cup	80	28%	2.5	1	12

Product and Portion Size	Calories	% Cal from Fat	Total Fat (g)	Bad Fat (g)	Net Carbs (g)
Del Monte, w/green beans & ham flavor, ½ cup	30	0%	0	0	5
Del Monte, new potatoes, sliced, ⅔ cup	60	0%	0	0	11
S&W, new potatoes, whole, 2 potatoes	60	0%	0	0	11
Frozen					
Birds Eye, baby whole potatoes, 7	80	0%	0	0	16
Birds Eye, roasted potatoes & broccoli, ⅔ cup	100	36%	4	2	14
Cascadian Farm, country style, ¾ cup	50	0%	0	0	11
Cascadian Farm, crinkle cut French fries, 18 pcs	130	27%	4	1	19
Cascadian Farm, hash browns, 1 cup	60	0%	0	0	13
Cascadian Farm, spud puppies, 10 pcs	160	60%	7	1.5	21
Cascadian Farm, wedge cut, 8 pcs	110	23%	2.5	0.5	19
McCain, crinkle cut, 3 oz	130	27%	4	0	19
McCain, golden crisp, 3 oz	150	40%	7	0.5	18
McCain, mash bites, 3 oz	170	35%	7	0.5	22
McCain Roasters, All-American, 3 oz	120	21%	3	0	19
McCain Roasters, French onion, 3 oz	110	23%	3	0	18
McCain Roasters, grilled garlic & onion, 3 oz	120	21%	3	0	20
McCain seasoned beer battered wedges, 3 oz	140	50%	7	4	15

Product and Portion Size	Calories	% Cal from Fat	Total Fat (g)	Bad Fat (g)	Net Carbs (g)
McCain seasoned spirals, 3 oz	140	43%	7	0.5	16
McCain seasoned wedges w/skin, 3 oz	120	38%	5	0	15
McCain shoestring, 45 pcs	210	33%	8	0.5	29
McCain steak fries, 8 pcs	120	33%	3	0	19
McCain Tasti Tater shaped, 8 pcs	160	38%	7	0.5	17
OreIda, golden crinkles, 3 oz	130	27%	4	2.5	15
OreIda, hash browns, ¾ cup	80	0%	0	0	16
OreIda, shoestring, 3 oz	150	33%	6	3	17
OreIda, steak fries, 3 oz	110	23%	3	1	17
Mixes/Boxed—Betty Crocker					
Au gratin, ½ cup	100	10%	1.5	1	20
Butter & herb mash, ½ cup	90	11%	1	1	17
Cheddar & bacon, ⅔ cup	100	15%	1.5	1	19
Delux cheesy cheddar, ⅔ cup	130	31%	4.5	2.5	20
Delux creamy scallop, ½ cup	140	29%	4.5	2.5	21
Delux 3 cheese mashed, ½ cup	150	30%	5	3.5	23
Hash browns, ½ cup	120	0%	0	0	24
Homestyle cheesey scalloped, ⅔ cup	100	15%	1.5	1	18

Product and Portion Size	Calories	% Cal from Fat	Total Fat (g)	Bad Fat (g)	Net Carbs (g)
Homestyle creamy butter mash, ½ cup	90	11%	1	1	18
Julienne, ⅓ cup	90	11%	1	0	18
Roasted garlic, ⅔ cup	90	17%	1.5	1	18
Specialty scalloped, ½ cup	90	11%	1	1	19
Specialty sour cream & chives, ⅔ cup	100	10%	1	0.5	19
Mixes/Boxed—Idahoan					
Mashed 4 cheese, ¼ cup mix	100	25%	2.5	1	18
Mashed herb & butter, ¼ cup mix	110	23%	2.5	1	18
Mashed homestyle, ¼ cup mix	110	18%	2.5	1	19
Mashed, original, ⅓ cup mix	80	0%	0	0	16
POTATO CHIPS					
Herr's					
Bacon & horseradish, 1 oz	160	56%	10	1.5	14
BBQ, 1 oz	150	60%	10	3	13
Honey mustard, 1 oz	150	60%	10	3	13
Ketchup, 1 oz	150	60%	10	2.5	14
Kettle-cooked, jalapeno, 1 oz	160	56%	10	2.5	13
Kettle-cooked, original, 1 oz	160	56%	10	2.5	13

Product and Portion Size	Calories	% Cal from Fat	Total Fat (g)	Bad Fat (g)	Net Carbs (g)
Pa Dutch style, 1 oz	150	60%	10	2.5	13
Sour cream & onion, 1 oz	150	60%	10	3	13
Sweet island, 1 oz	150	60%	10	3	21
Lay's					
Baked, cheddar & sour cream, 1 oz	120	21%	3	0.5	19
Baked, original crisps, 1 oz	110	14%	1.5	0	21
Baked, sour cream & onion, 1 oz	120	21%	3	0	21
Deli style, original, 1 oz	150	60%	10	3	15
Hot n spicy, BBQ flavor, 1 oz	150	60%	10	3	14
Kettle cooked, jalapeno, 1 oz	140	50%	8	1	15
Kettle cooked, mesquite BBQ, 1 oz	140	50%	8	1	15
Kettle cooked, original, 1 oz	150	53%	8	1	17
Lightly salted, 1 oz	150	60%	10	1	14
Natural thick cut country BBQ, 1 oz	150	53%	9	1	14
Stax, cheddar flavored, 1 oz	150	60%	10	2.5	14
Stax, Hidden Valley ranch, 1 oz	150	53%	9	2.5	14
Stax, original, 1 oz	160	56%	10	2.5	14
Stax, salt & vinegar, 1 oz	150	53%	9	2.5	13

Product and Portion Size	Calories	% Cal from Fat	Total Fat (g)	Bad Fat (g)	Net Carbs (g)
Wavy, au gratin, 1 oz	150	60%	10	3	13
Wavy, hickory BBQ, 1 oz	150	53%	9	1	15
Pringles					
Chili cheese, 1 oz	160	63%	11	3	12
Fat-free original, 1 oz	70	0%	0	0	13
Fat-free sour cream & onion, 1 oz	70	0%	0	0	13
Loaded baked potato, 1 oz	150	60%	10	3	13
Original, 1 oz	160	63%	11	3	14
Ranch, 1 oz	160	63%	11	3	12
Sour cream & onion, 1 oz	160	56%	10	1.5	14
Wise					
BBQ flavored, 1 oz	150	60%	10	3	14
Chipotle flavored, 1 oz	150	60%	10	2	13
Kettle cooked, jalapeno, 1 oz	140	50%	8	2.5	15
Kettle cooked, natural, 1 oz	150	53%	9	2.5	14
Original, flat cut, 1 oz	150	60%	10	3	14
PRETZELS					
Bachman					
Butter twists, 1 oz	110	9%	1	0	22

Product and Portion Size	Calories	% Cal from Fat	Total Fat (g)	Bad Fat (g)	Net Carbs (g)
Classic twist, 1 oz	100	10%	1	0	21
Nutzels, 1 oz	110	9%	1	0	22
Peanut butter pretzels, 1 oz	160	44%	8	1.5	14
Sourdough bites, 1 oz	110	9%	1	0	21
Wheat & honey pretzelmack, 1 oz	110	9%	1	0	22
Herr's					
Bite size hard, 1 oz	100	0%	0	0	21
Chocolate covered rods, 7/10 oz	90	22%	2.5	2	14
Extra dark specials, 1 oz	110	9%	1	0	19
Honey wheat, 1 oz	110	9%	2	0	19
Peanut butter filled, 10	160	44%	8	1.5	14
Specials, 1½ oz	170	9%	2	0	29
Quinlan					
Butter flavored braided twists, 1 oz	110	9%	1	0	22
Honey wheat braided twists, 1 oz	110	9%	1	0	23
Mini, 1 oz	110	9%	1	0	22
Sticks, f-f, 1 oz	100	0%	0	0	22

Product and Portion Size	Calories	% Cal from Fat	Total Fat (g)	Bad Fat (g)	Net Carbs (g)
Rold Gold					
Cheddar tiny twists, 1 oz	110	9%	1	0	21
Classic rods, 1 oz	110	9%	1	0	21
Classic thins, 1 oz	110	9%	1	0	22
Fat-free tiny twists, 1 oz	100	0%	0	0	22
Hard sourdough, 1 oz	100	5%	0.5	0	20
Honey mustard tiny twists, 1 oz	110	9%	1	0	22
Land O Lakes butter, 1 oz	110	14%	1.5	0	21
Snyder's of Hanover					
Butter snaps, 1 oz	120	8%	1	0	25
Carb fix nibblers, 1 oz	120	17%	2	0	21
Homestyle, 1 oz	120	8%	1	0	25
Honey wheat sticks, 1 oz	120	17%	2	0	24
Pretzel sesame sticks, 1 oz	120	13%	2	0	23
Sourdough hard, 1 oz	100	0%	0	0	22
12-grain sticks, 1 oz	120	17%	2	0	23
Superpretzel—Frozen					
Pretzelfils, mozzarella, 2	130	23%	3.5	1.5	19

Product and Portion Size	Calories	% Cal from Fat	Total Fat (g)	Bad Fat (g)	Net Carbs (g)
Pretzelfils, pepperjack, 2	130	23%	3.5	1.5	20
Pretzelfils, pizza, 2	130	15%	2	2	21
Soft pretzel, w/o added salt, 1	160	6%	1	0	33
Soft pretzel bites, 5 w/o added salt	150	3%	0.5	0	31
Softstix, 2	130	19%	3	1.5	21
PRUNES/PRUNE BEVERAGE					
Knudsen, juice, organic, 8 oz	170	0%	0	0	17
Old Orchard, juice cocktail, 8 oz	61	0%	0	0	11
Sunsweet bite size or whole, 1.5 oz	100	0%	0	0	21
Sunsweet ready to serve, ⅔ cup	150	0%	0	0	34
Sunsweet, juice w/ or w/o pulp, 8 oz	180	0%	0	0	40
PUDDING					
Handi-Snacks, banana or vanilla, 3.5 oz	90	11%	1	0	20
Handi-Snacks, chocolate, 3.5 oz	100	10%	1	1	22
Handi-Snacks, chocolate, f-f, 3.5 oz	90	0%	0	0	21
Handi-Snacks, double fudge, rocky road, 3.5 oz	100	10%	1	1	22
Handi-Snacks, rice, 3.5 oz	140	35%	6	1	19

Product and Portion Size	Calories	% Cal from Fat	Total Fat (g)	Bad Fat (g)	Net Carbs (g)
Jell-O					
Banana cream, cook & serve, ½ cup	80	0%	0	0	20
Banana cream, instant, ½ cup	90	0%	0	0	23
Butterscotch, instant, ½ cup	90	0%	0	0	23
Cheesecake, instant, ½ cup	100	0%	0	0	24
Chocolate, cook & serve, ½ cup	90	0%	0	0	21
Chocolate, cook & serve, sugar free, ½ cup	30	0%	0	0	6
Chocolate fudge, sugar & fat-free, ½ cup	30	0%	0	0	7
Coconut cream, cook & serve, ½ cup	90	22%	2.5	2.5	17
Lemon, instant, ½ cup	90	0%	0	0	24
Mixed berry, Smoothie Snack, 1 serv.	100	25%	2.5	1.5	18
Oreo cookies 'n cream, ½ cup	120	8%	1	0	28
Pistachio, instant, ½ cup	100	0%	0.5	0	23
Strawberry banana, Smoothie Snack, 1 serv.	100	25%	2.5	1.5	18
Vanilla, cook & serve, ½ cup	80	0%	0	0	20
Jell-O Pudding Snacks					
Caramel, sugar free, 4 oz	60	16%	1	1	13
Chocolate, 4 oz	140	25%	4	1.5	26

Product and Portion Size	Calories	% Cal from Fat	Total Fat (g)	Bad Fat (g)	Net Carbs (g)
Chocolate, f-f, 4 oz	100	0%	0	0	22
Chocolate vanilla swirl, 4 oz	140	25%	4	1.5	25
Oreo, 4 oz	140	25%	4	1.5	26
Strawberry & crème, 4 oz	130	19%	3	1	25
Tapioca, 4 oz	130	19%	3	1	25
Vanilla caramel, f-f, 4 oz	100	0%	0	0	23
Uncle Ben's					
Cinnamon & raisin rice pudding, ½ cup prep.	160	6%	1	0	37
French vanilla, ½ cup prep.	120	0%	0	0	27
PUMPKIN					
Fresh, cooked, no salt, mashed, 1 cup	49	3%	0	0	9
Libby's canned, 100% pure, ½ cup	40	13%	0.5	0	4
Libby's canned, pie mix, ⅓ cup	90	5%	0.5	0	17
Seeds, kernels, roasted, no salt, 1 oz	**147**	**68%**	**12**	**2**	**3**
Seeds, whole, roasted, no salt, 1 oz	**126**	**36%**	**5**	**1**	**15**
PUNCH					
Capri Sun: fruit punch, grape, orange, pacific cooler, red berry, 200 ml	100	0%	0	0	27

Product and Portion Size	Calories	% Cal from Fat	Total Fat (g)	Bad Fat (g)	Net Carbs (g)
Capri Sun, splash cooler, strawberry, tropical punch, 200 ml	90	0%	0	0	25
Hi-C: Crazy Citrus, Flashin' Fruit, Orange Lavaburst, 200 ml box	90	0%	0	0	25
Hi-C: Boppin' Strawberry, Poppin' Lemonade, Strawberry Kiwi, 200 ml box	100	0%	0	0	27
Hi-C Blast					
Berry Blue, 8 oz	120	0%	0	0	32
Blue watermelon, Fruit punch, Wild berry, 200 ml pouch	100	0%	0	0	26
Fruit Pow, 1 bottle	180	0%	0	0	46
Orange, 200 ml pouch	90	0%	0	0	25
Raspberry kiwi, strawberry, 200 ml pouch	100	0%	0	0	27
Kool-Aid bursts, tropical punch, 200 ml	100	0%	0	0	24
Kool-Aid Mix, tropical punch, 8 oz	60	0%	0	0	16
Minute Maid, berry, citrus, grape, 8 oz	120	0%	0	0	32
Minute Maid, tropical, 8 oz	110	0%	0	0	30
Tropicana 100% juice fruit punch, 10 oz	170	0%	0	0	40

Product and Portion Size	Calories	% Cal from Fat	Total Fat (g)	Bad Fat (g)	Net Carbs (g)
RADISHES, raw, ½ cup slices	9	5%	0	0	1
RAISINS					
Dole, ¼ cup	130	0%	0	0	29
Sun-Maid, baking, ¼ cup	110	0%	0	0	25
Sun-Maid, chocolate covered, 30 pcs	170	35%	6	4	24
Sun-Maid, chocolate yogurt, ¼ cup	120	33%	4	3.5	21
Sun-Maid, golden or regular, ¼ cup	130	0%	0	0	29
Sun-Maid, vanilla yogurt, ¼ cup	130	35%	5	4	20
RASPBERRIES, raw, red, 1 cup	64	10%	1	0	7
Cascadian Farm, organic, frozen, 1¼ cup	70	7%	1	0	9
RED BEANS					
Eden Foods, organic, canned, ½ cup	100	5%	0.5	0	12
S&W, canned, Louisiana style, ½ cup	80	0%	0	0	15
RED SNAPPER, broiled, 3 oz	109	12%	1	0	0
REFRIED BEANS					
Eden Foods					
Black beans, organic, ½ cup	110	10%	1.5	0	11
Kidney beans, organic, ½ cup	80	10%	1	0	9

Product and Portion Size	Calories	% Cal from Fat	Total Fat (g)	Bad Fat (g)	Net Carbs (g)
Pinto, organic, ½ cup	90	10%	1	0	12
Pinto, spicy, organic, ½ cup	90	10%	1	0	12
Old El Paso					
Fat-free, ½ cup	100	0%	0	0	12
Fat-free, spicy, ½ cup	100	0%	0	0	12
Traditional, ½ cup	100	5%	0.5	0	11
Vegetarian, ½ cup	100	10%	1	0	11
w/sausage, ½ cup	200	60%	13	5	10
Taco Bell					
Original, f-f, ½ cup	110	0%	0	0	15
Vegetarian, ½ cup	140	18%	3	0.5	16
RELISH					
Claussen, sweet, 1 Tbs	15	0%	0	0	3
Vlasic, dill, 1 Tbs	5	0%	0	0	1
Vlasic, relish mixers, 1 Tbs	10	0%	0	0	2
Vlasic, specialty blend, 1 Tbs	20	0%	0	0	5
Vlasic, sweet, 1 Tbs	15	0%	0	0	4
RHUBARB, raw, diced, ⅔ cup	26	0%	0	0	2
Frozen (Dole), 1 cup	30	0%	0	0	4

Product and Portion Size	Calories	% Cal from Fat	Total Fat (g)	Bad Fat (g)	Net Carbs (g)
RICE					
Long grain, 1 cup prep.	194	3%	1	0	40
Medium or short grain, 1 cup prep.	242	1%	0	0	52
Carolina, extra long grain white, ¾ cup prep.	150	0%	0	0	35
Carolina, gold (parboiled), 1 cup prep.	160	0%	0	0	36
Carolina, jasmine, ¾ cup prep.	160	0%	0	0	36
Carolina, long grain brown, ¾ cup prep.	150	6%	1	0	31
Minute Rice, instant long grain brown, ¾ cup prep.	170	9%	1.5	0	32
Minute Rice, instant long grain white, ¾ cup prep.	160	0%	0	0	35
Uncle Ben's fast & natural brown, 1 cup prep.	190	8%	1.5	0	40
Uncle Ben's instant white, 1 cup prep.	190	3%	0.5	0	42
Uncle Ben's long grain & wild, 1 cup prep.	240	13%	3.5	0	43
RICE MIXES					
Betty Crocker Bowl Appetit					
Cheddar broccoli rice, 1 bowl	290	21%	7	4.5	49
Herb chicken vegetable, 1 bowl	260	17%	5	2.5	47
Teriyaki rice, 1 bowl	260	10%	3	1.5	52

Product and Portion Size	Calories	% Cal from Fat	Total Fat (g)	Bad Fat (g)	Net Carbs (g)
Carolina					
Authentic Spanish, ⅓ cup mix	180	3%	0	0	41
Black bean & rice, ⅓ cup mix	200	7%	1.5	0	34
Chicken & rice, ⅓ cup mix	190	3%	0	0	41
Classic pilaf, ⅓ cup mix	190	0%	0	0	42
Saffron yellow, ⅓ cup mix	190	0%	0	0	42
Spicy yellow, ⅓ cup mix	180	3%	0.5	0	40
Knorr-Lipton					
Beef, ½ cup mix	230	0%	0.5	0	48
Cajun style, dirty rice, ½ cup mix	250	6%	1.5	0	48
Cajun style, garlic butter, ½ cup mix	260	13%	4	2	47
Cajun style, New Orleans, ½ cup mix	250	6%	1.5	0	48
Cajun style, red rice & beans, ½ cup mix	290	3%	1	0	55
Cheddar broccoli, ½ cup mix	230	7%	1.5	0.5	45
Chicken broccoli, ½ cup mix	220	5%	1	0	43
Herb & butter, ½ cup mix	250	16%	4.5	2.5	45
Rice medley, ½ cup mix	210	5%	1	0	42
Rice pilaf, ½ cup mix	220	9%	2	0	42

Product and Portion Size	Calories	% Cal from Fat	Total Fat (g)	Bad Fat (g)	Net Carbs (g)
Near East					
Brown rice pilaf, ¼ cup mix	180	6%	1	0	38
Long grain & wild, ⅓ cup mix	190	0%	0.5	0	41
Rice pilaf toasted almond, ¼ cup mix	200	12%	3	0	38
Sundried tomato & basil, ⅓ cup mix	240	2%	0.5	0	52
Rice-A-Roni					
Beef, ⅓ cup mix	230	4%	1	0	48
Broccoli au gratin, ⅓ cup mix	260	19%	6	3	44
Cheesy Italian herb, ⅓ cup mix	260	19%	6	2	44
Chicken, ⅓ cup mix	230	4%	1	0	49
Chicken & garlic, ⅓ cup mix	190	0%	0.5	0	39
Fried, ⅓ cup mix	240	6%	1.5	0	47
Herb & butter, ⅓ cup mix	240	6%	1.5	0.5	51
Pilaf, ⅓ cup mix	230	4%	1	0	49
Spanish, ⅓ cup mix	180	0%	0.5	0	38
RICE BEVERAGES					
Rice Dream, carob, 8 oz	150	17%	2.5	0	32
Rice Dream, chocolate enriched, 8 oz	170	18%	3	0	36

Product and Portion Size	Calories	% Cal from Fat	Total Fat (g)	Bad Fat (g)	Net Carbs (g)
Rice Dream, original, 8 oz	120	17%	2	0	25
Rice Dream, vanilla, 8 oz	130	15%	2	0	28
Rice Dream, vanilla heartwise, 8 oz	140	14%	2	0	27
Westbrae, plain, 8 oz	100	25%	2.5	0	18
Westbrae, vanilla, 8 oz	120	21%	2.5	0	22
RICE CAKES/CRACKERS/CHIPS					
Eden Foods					
Brown rice chips, 25 chips	150	47%	7	1.5	19
Brown rice crackers, 8	120	13%	2	0	20
Nori maki rice crackers, 15	110	0%	0	0	22
Quaker Rice Cakes					
Apple cinnamon, 1	50	0%	0	0	11
Butter popped corn, 1	35	0%	0	0	8
Chocolate crunch, 1	60	16%	1	0	12
Peanut butter chocolate chip, 1	60	16%	1	0	12
White cheddar, 1	45	12%	0.5	0	8
RICE PUDDING; see "Pudding"					
ROCKFISH, Pacific, baked, 3 oz	103	15%	2	0	14

Product and Portion Size	Calories	% Cal from Fat	Total Fat (g)	Bad Fat (g)	Net Carbs (g)
ROLLS (nonsweet)					
Pepperidge Farm					
Carb style, hamburger, 1	110	9%	1	0	14
Farmhouse country wheat, 1	220	18%	4.5	1	35
Frankfurter, 1	140	16%	2.5	1	23
Hamburger, 1	120	15%	2	0.5	21
Hot & crusty French, 1	100	9%	1	0	18
Hot & crusty 7 grain, 1	110	16%	2	0.5	19
Onion sandwich bun, 1	150	15%	2.5	0.5	27
Parker house dinner, 1	80	23%	2	0.5	13
Soft 100% whole wheat Kaiser, 1	200	11%	2.5	1	32
Soft country style dinner, 1	90	15%	1.5	0	16
Soft hoagie, 1	210	26%	6	1.5	33
Soft white Kaiser, 1	210	11%	2.5	0.5	36
Pillsbury					
Crescent big & buttery, 1	170	53%	10	5	19
Crescent big & flaky, 1	180	50%	10	5	19
Crescent butterflake, 1	110	55%	6	3.5	11

Product and Portion Size	Calories	% Cal from Fat	Total Fat (g)	Bad Fat (g)	Net Carbs (g)
Crescent original, 1	110	55%	6	3.5	11
Dinner, white quick, 1	110	18%	2	1	17
Freezer to Microwave, white dinner, 1	150	23%	4	2	25
Freezer to Oven crusty French, 1	100	10%	1.5	0	17
Freezer to Oven, dinner, garlic, 1	140	43%	6	2.5	16
Freezer to Oven, dinner, whole wheat, 1	90	11%	1	0	14
Sara Lee					
Classic heart healthy wheat hamburger, 1	190	13%	2.5	0.5	34
Classic wheat buns, 1	200	15%	3.5	1	35
Classic white buns, 1	200	13%	3	1	36
Gourmet hot dog, 1	120	13%	1.5	0	22
ROLLS (Sweet)—Pillsbury					
Freezer to Oven sweet, cinnamon, 1	290	31%	10	5	45
Grands! Extra rich cinnamon w/icing, 1	320	28%	10	5.5	53
Grands! Sweet cinnamon w/icing, 1	310	26%	9	4.5	53
Grands! Sweet cinnamon w/icing, reduced fat, 1	300	20%	6	3	55
Grands! Sweet orange, 1	330	30%	11	5.5	52
Sweet Rolls, caramel, 1	170	35%	7	4	23

Product and Portion Size	Calories	% Cal from Fat	Total Fat (g)	Bad Fat (g)	Net Carbs (g)
Sweet Rolls, cinnamon w/cream cheese icing, 1	150	33%	5	3.5	22
Sweet Rolls, cinnamon raisin w/icing, 1	170	35%	6	3.5	25
Sweet Rolls, cinnamon w/icing, 1	150	30%	5	3.5	22
Sweet Rolls, cinnamon w/icing, sugar free, 1	110	27%	3.5	2	20
Sweet Rolls, golden homestyle cinnamon, 1	130	23%	3	2	23
Sweet Rolls, orange w/icing, 1	170	35%	7	3.5	24
SALAD DRESSING					
Annie's Naturals					
Artichoke parmesan, 2 Tbs	130	92%	13	1.5	1
Balsamic vinaigrette, 2 Tbs	100	90%	10	0.5	3
Thousand island, 2 Tbs	90	67%	7	1	5
Woodstock, 2 Tbs	110	91%	11	1	1
Kraft					
Catalina, f-f, 2 Tbs	35	0%	0	0	7
Creamy French, 2 Tbs	160	88%	15	2.5	5
Creamy Italian, 2 Tbs	110	91%	11	1.5	2
Italian, f-f, 2 Tbs	15	0%	0	0	4
Ranch, 2 Tbs	170	100%	18	3	2

Product and Portion Size	Calories	% Cal from Fat	Total Fat (g)	Bad Fat (g)	Net Carbs (g)
Ranch garlic, 2 Tbs	180	94%	19	3	1
Roka blue cheese, 2 Tbs	130	92%	13	2.5	1
Thousand island, 2 Tbs	120	75%	10	1.5	0
Three cheese Italian, 2 Tbs	130	100%	14	2.5	1
Zesty Italian, 2 Tbs	110	91%	11	1.5	2
Kraft—Carb Well					
Classic Caesar, 1 Tbs	110	91%	11	2	0
Creamy French, 2 Tbs	100	100%	11	1.5	0
Italian, 2 Tbs	70	100%	10	1	0
Light buttermilk ranch, 2 Tbs	60	83%	6	1	0
Light Italian, 2 Tbs	20	75%	1.5	0	0
Ranch, 2 Tbs	110	91%	11	1.5	0
Roka blue cheese, 2 Tbs	120	100%	13	2	0
Kraft—Light Done Right					
Creamy French, 2 Tbs	80	50%	4.5	0.5	9
Italian, 2 Tbs	40	75%	3	0.5	3
Ranch, 2 Tbs	80	75%	7	0.5	3
Roka blue, 2 Tbs	70	86%	6	1	3
Zesty Italian, reduced fat, 2 Tbs	25	60%	1.5	0	2

Product and Portion Size	Calories	% Cal from Fat	Total Fat (g)	Bad Fat (g)	Net Carbs (g)
Kraft—Special Collection					
Caesar Italian w/oregano, 2 Tbs	100	90%	10	1.5	2
Creamy poppyseed, 2 Tbs	130	69%	10	2	8
Greek vinaigrette, 2 Tbs	110	91%	11	1.5	25
Italian Pesto, 2 Tbs	70	64%	5	0.5	5
Italian vinaigrette, 2 Tbs	50	70%	4	0	4
Sun dried tomato, 2 Tbs	60	75%	5	0.5	4
Tangy tomato bacon, 2 Tbs	130	69%	10	1.5	8
Newman's Own					
Caesar, 2 Tbs	150	93%	15	2	2
Olive oil & vinegar, 2 Tbs	150	96%	16	2.5	1
Ranch, 2 Tbs	140	93%	15	2	2
2000 island, 2 Tbs	140	86%	14	2	2
Three cheese balsamic, 2 Tbs	100	100%	11	1.5	2
Seven Seas					
Creamy Italian, 2 Tbs	110	100%	12	2	2
Green goddess, 2 Tbs	130	95%	13	2	1
Red wine vinaigrette, 2 Tbs	90	89%	9	0.5	2

Product and Portion Size	Calories	% Cal from Fat	Total Fat (g)	Bad Fat (g)	Net Carbs (g)
Viva Italian, 2 Tbs	90	89%	9	0.5	2
Viva Italian, reduced fat, 2 Tbs	45	78%	4	0.5	2
South Beach Diet					
Italian w/extra olive oil, 2 Tbs	60	67%	4.5	0	3
Ranch, 2 Tbs	70	86%	7	1	2
Wishbone					
Chunky blue cheese, 2 Tbs	150	93%	15	2.5	2
Creamy Caesar, 2 Tbs	170	94%	18	3	1
Delux French, 2 Tbs	120	83%	11	1.5	5
Garlic ranch, 2 Tbs	140	100%	15	2	2
Russian, 2 Tbs	120	42%	6	1	14
Sweet 'n spicy, 2 Tbs	130	85%	12	2	6
Thousand island, 2 Tbs	130	85%	12	2	5
Wishbone—Fat Free					
Chunky blue cheese, 2 Tbs	35	0%	0	0	5
Italian, 2 Tbs	20	0%	0	0	4
Ranch, 2 Tbs	30	0%	0	0	7

Product and Portion Size	Calories	% Cal from Fat	Total Fat (g)	Bad Fat (g)	Net Carbs (g)
Wishbone—Just2Good					
Blue cheese, 2 Tbs	50	40%	2	0.5	6
Creamy Caesar, 2 Tbs	50	40%	2	0.5	7
Deluxe French, 2 Tbs	50	40%	2	0	7
Honey Dijon, 2 Tbs	50	40%	2	0	7
Ranch, 2 Tbs	40	50%	2	0	5
Thousand island, 2 Tbs	50	40%	2	0	9
Wishbone—Salad Spritzers					
Balsamic breeze, 10 sprays	10	100%	1	0	1
Italian vinaigrette, 10 sprays	10	100%	1	0	1
Red wine mist, 10 sprays	10	100%	1	0	1
Wishbone—Western					
With bacon flavor, 2 Tbs	140	71%	11	1.5	10
With blue cheese, 2 Tbs	140	79%	12	2	9
Fat-free, 2 Tbs	50	0%	0	0	12
Original, 2 Tbs	160	69%	12	1.5	11
SALAMI					
Hebrew National, beef, 3 slices	150	80%	13	6	0

Product and Portion Size	Calories	% Cal from Fat	Total Fat (g)	Bad Fat (g)	Net Carbs (g)
Oscar Mayer, cotto, 1 oz	70	71%	6	2	1
Oscar Mayer, cotto beef, 1 oz	60	67%	4.5	2	1
Oscar Mayer, hard, 1 oz	100	70%	8	3	1
SALMON					
Canned, blueback (Bumblebee), 2.2 oz	**110**	**55%**	**7**	**1.5**	**0**
Canned, keta (Bumblebee), 2.2 oz	**90**	**39%**	**4**	**1**	**0**
Canned, pink (Bumblebee), 2.2 oz	**90**	**50%**	**5**	**1**	**0**
Canned, red (Bumblebee), 2.2 oz	**110**	**55%**	**7**	**1.5**	**0**
Canned, pink (Chicken of the Sea), 2 oz	**60**	**33%**	**2**	**1**	**0**
Canned, trad. red (Chicken of the Sea), ¼ cup	**110**	**55%**	**7**	**3**	**0**
Fresh, Atlantic wild, cooked dry, 3 oz	**155**	**40%**	**7**	**1**	**0**
Fresh, Chinook wild, cooked dry, 3 oz	**196**	**52%**	**11**	**3**	**0**
Smoked Pacific (Chicken of the Sea), 1 pkg	**120**	**25%**	**3.5**	**1**	**1**
Steak w/orange glaze (Chicken of the Sea), 1 pkg	**170**	**9%**	**1.5**	**0.5**	**12**
SALSA					
Muir Glen organic, black bean & corn, 2 Tbs	20	0%	0	0	4
Muir Glen organic, mild, 2 Tbs	10	0%	0	0	3
Newman's Own, black bean & corn, 2 Tbs	20	0%	0	0	5

Product and Portion Size	Calories	% Cal from Fat	Total Fat (g)	Bad Fat (g)	Net Carbs (g)
Newman's Own, mango, 2 Tbs	20	0%	0	0	5
Newman's Own, natural bandito mild, 2 Tbs	10	0%	0	0	2
Newman's Own, peach, 2 Tbs	25	0%	0	0	5
Newman's Own, tequila lime, 2 Tbs	15	0%	0	0	3
Old El Paso, cheese 'n salsa medium, 2 Tbs	40	63%	3	1	3
Old El Paso, thick 'n chunky, mild, 2 Tbs	10	0%	0	0	3
Pace, chunky, 2 Tbs	10	0%	0	0	1
Pace, lime & garlic chunky, 2 Tbs	15	0%	0	0	2
Taco Bell, salsa con queso, 2 Tbs	40	63%	3	0.5	3
Taco Bell, thick 'n chunky, mild, 2 Tbs	15	0%	0	0	3
SARDINES					
Bumblebee, in mustard, 3.75 oz	**130**	**46%**	**6**	**1.5**	**0**
Bumblebee, in soya oil, 3.75 oz	**130**	**62%**	**9**	**2**	**0**
Bumblebee, in water, 3.75 oz	**120**	**58%**	**7**	**2**	**0**
Chicken of the Sea, smoked, in oil, 1 can	**190**	**68%**	**14**	**6**	**2**
Chicken of the Sea, in tomato, 1 can	**130**	**38%**	**6**	**2**	**0**
Chicken of the Sea, in water, 1 can	**100**	**40%**	**4**	**2**	**2**
Crown Prince, brisling in mustard, 1 can	**210**	**71%**	**16**	**6**	**<1**

Product and Portion Size	Calories	% Cal from Fat	Total Fat (g)	Bad Fat (g)	Net Carbs (g)
Crown Prince, brisling in soy oil, 1 can	200	70%	16	4.5	0
Crown Prince, brisling in tomato, 1 can	210	71%	16	6	0
SAUCES					
A1 Sauce					
Jamaican jerk steak sauce, 2 Tbs	25	20%	0.5	0	5
New York steak sauce, 2 Tbs	20	0%	0	0	5
Teriyaki steak sauce, 2 Tbs	20	0%	0	0	5
Eden Foods					
Shoyu soy sauce, 1 Tbs	15	0%	0	0	2
Tamari soy sauce, 1 Tbs	10	0%	0	0	2
Kraft					
Cocktail, 2 Tbs	60	8%	0.5	0	10
Coleslaw maker, 2 Tbs	110	72%	9	1.5	7
Sweet & sour, 2 Tbs	60	0%	0	0	13
Tartar sauce, 2 Tbs	70	70%	6	1	4
Old El Paso					
Enchilada, mild, ¼ cup	25	40%	1	0	3
Taco sauce, mild, 1 Tbs	5	0%	0	0	1
Zesty ranch sauce, 2 Tbs	70	85%	6	1	2

Product and Portion Size	Calories	% Cal from Fat	Total Fat (g)	Bad Fat (g)	Net Carbs (g)
SAUERKRAUT					
Del Monte, 2 Tbs	0	0%	0	0	0
Del Monte, Bavarian, 2 Tbs	15	0%	0	0	4
Eden, organic, ½ cup	25	0%	0	0	4
S&W, 2 Tbs	0	0%	0	0	1
SAUSAGE					
Armour					
Brown & serve, bacon flavor, 3 links	180	78%	16	6	2
Brown & serve, beef, 3 links	230	87%	22	10	1
Brown & serve, country recipe, 3 links	210	81%	19	7	2
Brown & serve, lite original, 3 links	120	67%	8	3	3
Brown & serve, turkey, 3 links	120	67%	8	2.5	2
Chicken Vienna sausage, 3 links	90	66%	7	2	1
Bob Evans					
Pork sausage links, maple, 2 links	130	77%	11	4	2
Pork sausage links, original, 2 links	130	67%	10	4	0
Hillshire					
Smoked, beef, 2 oz	190	79%	17	8	3

Product and Portion Size	Calories	% Cal from Fat	Total Fat (g)	Bad Fat (g)	Net Carbs (g)
Smoked, brat, 1 link	240	79%	21	8	3
Jimmy Dean					
Pork sausage link, original, 3 links	260	81%	24	8	2
Pork sausage, maple patties, 2 patties	260	81%	23	8	6
Libby, Vienna, 3 links	130	85%	12	5	0
Lightlife (soy)					
Gimme lean sausage style, 2 oz	50	0%	0	0	2
Smart brats, 1 link	120	45%	5	0	4
Smart links country breakfast, 2 links	100	31%	3.5	0.5	4
Louis Rich, turkey sausage, 3 oz	120	58%	8	2.5	1
Oscar Mayer					
Pork sausage links, 2 links	130	77%	11	4	1
Pork sausage patties, 2 patties	180	72%	15	6	2
SCALLIONS, fresh, chopped, 1 cup	32	5%	0	0	4
SCALLOPS, bay or sea, 1 oz	**32**	**11%**	**0**	**0**	**15**
Mrs. Paul's fried breaded scallops, 13 pcs	260	38%	11	4	28
SESAME					
Arrowhead Mills, tahini (sesame spread), 2 Tbs	**190**	**84%**	**18**	**2.5**	**2**
Maranatha tahini butter, no salt, 2 Tbs	**190**	**74%**	**16**	**2**	**7**

Product and Portion Size	Calories	% Cal from Fat	Total Fat (g)	Bad Fat (g)	Net Carbs (g)
SHAD, American, cooked dry, 3 oz	214	63%	15	0	0
SHERBET					
Breyers, orange, ½ cup	130	12%	1.5	1	28
Breyers, rainbow, ½ cup	130	12%	1.5	1	27
Dreyer's, berry rainbow or tropical rainbow, ½ cup	130	12%	1.5	0.5	29
Dreyer's, key lime, ½ cup	130	12%	1.5	0.5	28
Dreyer's, orange cream, ½ cup	120	17%	2	1	23
Dreyer's, raspberry or strawberry, ½ cup	130	8%	1	0.5	28
Dreyer's, swiss orange, ½ cup	150	17%	3	2.5	30
SHRIMP					
Canned, regular (Bumblebee), ¼ cup	40	0%	0	0	0
Frozen, premium, cooked (Chicken of the Sea), 3 oz	80	12%	1	0	0
Frozen, premium, raw (Chicken of the Sea), 4 oz	120	12%	2	0	1
SNACK MIX					
Chex, bold party blend, ½ cup	140	37%	6	1.5	19
Chex mix, cheddar, ⅔ cup	130	27%	4	1	21
Chex mix, honey nut, ½ cup	130	27%	4	0.6	22
Chex mix, hot 'n spicy, ⅔ cup	130	27%	4	1.5	21

Product and Portion Size	Calories	% Cal from Fat	Total Fat (g)	Bad Fat (g)	Net Carbs (g)
Chex mix, peanut lovers, ½ cup	140	37%	6	1	18
Chex mix, summer ranch, ⅔ cup	120	21%	3	0.5	20
Chex mix, traditional, ⅔ cup	130	27%	4	0.5	21
Chex trail, ½ cup	140	29%	4.5	1.5	21
Chocolate peanut butter, ⅔ cup	150	30%	5	1.5	22
Chocolate turtle, ⅔ cup	150	30%	5	2	22
Eden Foods, all mixed up, 3 Tbs	160	69%	12	2	3
Gardetto's Italian cheese blend, ½ cup	140	32%	5	2	19
Gardetto's mustard pretzel mix, ½ cup	130	15%	2	0	23
Gardetto's snack mix, original, ½ cup	150	40%	6	3	19
Gardetto's snack mix, original, reduced fat, ½ cup	130	27%	4	2	19
Nabisco, cheddar, 1 oz	130	31%	4.5	1	18
Nabisco, traditional, 1 oz	130	35%	5	1	20
Planters, trail mix, fruit & nut, 1 oz	140	57%	9	2.5	12
Planter's trail mix, golden nut crunch, 1 oz	160	63%	11	2	10
Planter's trail mix, mixed nuts & raisins, 1 oz	150	67%	11	1.5	8
Planter's trail mix, nut & chocolate, 1 oz	160	56%	10	2.5	14
Planter's trail mix, spicy nuts, 1 oz	150	60%	10	1.5	11

Product and Portion Size	Calories	% Cal from Fat	Total Fat (g)	Bad Fat (g)	Net Carbs (g)
SOFT DRINKS					
Canada Dry					
Club soda, 8 oz	0	0%	0	0	0
Ginger ale, 8 oz	120	0%	0	0	33
Tonic water, 8 oz	90	0%	0	0	24
Dr. Pepper					
Berries & cream, 8 oz	100	0%	0	0	NA
Cherry vanilla, 8 oz	100	0%	0	0	NA
Original, 8 oz	100	0%	0	0	NA
Fresca, all flavors	0	0%	0	0	NA
Hansen's Natural Sodas					
Black cherry, grapefruit, orange mango, raspberry, vanilla cola, 12 oz	160	0%	0	0	44
Key lime, mandarin lime, 12 oz	130	0%	0	0	37
IBC					
Black cherry, 12 oz	180	0%	0	0	48
Cream, 12 oz	180	0%	0	0	48
Root beer, 12 oz	160	0%	0	0	43

Product and Portion Size	Calories	% Cal from Fat	Total Fat (g)	Bad Fat (g)	Net Carbs (g)
Mountain Dew					
Amp, 8 oz	110	0%	0	0	30
Baja blast, 8 oz	110	0%	0	0	30
Code red, 8 oz	110	0%	0	0	31
Livewire, 8 oz	110	0%	0	0	31
MDX, 8 oz	120	0%	0	0	33
Regular and caffeine free, 8 oz	110	0%	0	0	31
Pepsi					
Diet, all, 8 oz	0	0%	0	0	0
Regular and caffeine free, 8 oz	100	0%	0	0	27
Twist, 8 oz	100	0%	0	0	28
Wild cherry, 8 oz	110	0%	0	0	29
Vanilla, 8 oz	110	0%	0	0	28
Schweppes					
Club soda, 8 oz	0	0%	0	0	0
Ginger ale, 8 oz	80	0%	0	0	23
Ginger ale, diet, 8 oz	0	0%	0	0	0
Ginger ale, diet, grape, 0	0	0%	0	0	0
Tonic water, 8 oz	80	0%	0	0	23

Product and Portion Size	Calories	% Cal from Fat	Total Fat (g)	Bad Fat (g)	Net Carbs (g)
Sierra Mist					
Free, 8 oz	0	0%	0	0	0
Regular, 8 oz	100	0%	0	0	26
SOLE, cooked dry heat, 3 oz	99	12%	1	0	0
SORBET					
Ben 'N Jerry's					
Berried Treasure, ½ cup	110	0%	0	0	28
Jamaican Me Crazy, ½ cup	130	0%	0	0	28
Strawberry kiwi, ½ cup	110	0%	0	0	27
Haagen-Dazs					
Chocolate, ½ cup	130	45%	0.5	0	28
Mango, ½ cup	120	0%	0	0	37
Strawberry, ½ cup	120	0%	0	0	29
Tropical, ½ cup	150	0%	0	0	28
Zesty lemon, ½ cup	110	0%	0	0	28
SOUPS—Canned					
Campbell's					
Bean w/bacon, ½ cup	170	21%	4	1.5	17

Product and Portion Size	Calories	% Cal from Fat	Total Fat (g)	Bad Fat (g)	Net Carbs (g)
Beef noodle, ½ cup	70	32%	2.5	0.5	8
Beef w/vegetables & barley, ½ cup	90	15%	1.5	1	12
Black bean, ½ cup	110	12%	1.5	0.5	12
Broccoli cheese, ½ cup	100	41%	4.5	2	7
Chicken & dumplings, ½ cup	80	34%	3	1	9
Chicken & stars, ½ cup	70	26%	2	0.5	9
Chicken gumbo, ½ cup	60	15%	1	0.5	9
Chicken noodle, ½ cup	60	23%	1.5	0.5	7
Chicken vegetable, ½ cup	80	11%	1	0.5	13
Chicken won ton, ½ cup	60	15%	1	0.5	8
Cream of broccoli, 98% fat free, ½ cup	70	26%	2	0.5	8
Cream of celery, ½ cup	90	60%	6	0.5	6
Cream of chicken, ½ cup	120	60%	8	2.5	8
Cream of chicken, 98% fat free, ½ cup	70	32%	2.5	1	9
Cream of mushroom, ½ cup	100	56%	6	1.5	7
Cream of potato, ½ cup	90	20%	2	2	13
Cream of shrimp, ½ cup	90	60%	6	2	7
Creamy tomato ranchero, ½ cup	130	42%	6	2	12

Product and Portion Size	Calories	% Cal from Fat	Total Fat (g)	Bad Fat (g)	Net Carbs (g)
Fiesta chili beef, ½ cup	170	26%	5	2	17
Fiesta nacho cheese, ½ cup	120	60%	8	3	9
French onion, ½ cup	45	30%	1.5	1	5
Golden mushroom, ½ cup	80	39%	3.5	1	9
Goldfish meatball, ½ cup	80	28%	2.5	1.5	9
Green pea, ½ cup	180	15%	3	1	24
Hearty vegetable w/pasta, ½ cup	90	5%	0.5	0	17
Manhattan clam chowder, ½ cup	70	6%	0.5	0.5	10
Minestrone, ½ cup	90	10%	1	0.5	14
New England clam chowder, ½ cup	90	25%	2.5	0.5	12
New England clam chowder, 98% fat free, ½ cup	80	23%	2	0.5	12
Old fashioned vegetable, ½ cup	80	17%	1.5	0.5	12
Pepper pot, ½ cup	90	40%	4	1.5	8
Scotch broth, ½ cup	70	26%	2	1	7
SW style queso, ½ cup	150	42%	7	2.5	14
Split pea w/ham & bacon, ½ cup	180	18%	3.5	2	22
Tomato noodle, ½ cup	120	4%	0.5	0	23
Tomato, ½ cup	90	0%	0	0	19

Product and Portion Size	Calories	% Cal from Fat	Total Fat (g)	Bad Fat (g)	Net Carbs (g)
Vegetable beef, ½ cup	80	11%	1	0.5	12
Vegetarian vegetable, ½ cup	90	6%	0.5	0	16
Campbell's Chunky					
Baked potato w/cheddar & bacon, 1 cup	160	28%	5	2.5	20
Baked potato w/steak & cheese, 1 cup	210	43%	10	2.5	18
Beef w/country vegetable, 1 cup	150	15%	2.5	1	17
Cheese tortellini w/chicken & vegetables, 1 cup	110	16%	2	1	16
Chicken & dumplings, 1 cup	180	35%	7	2	15
Chicken mushroom chowder, 1 cup	210	51%	12	3	16
Grilled chicken & sausage gumbo, 1 cup	140	16%	2.5	1	18
Hearty bean & ham, 1 cup	180	10%	2	0.5	22
Hearty beef barley, 1 cup	170	13%	2.5	1	22
Honey roasted ham w/potatoes, 1 cup	130	17%	2.5	1	17
New England clam chowder, 1 cup	190	43%	9	2	19
Pepper steak, 1 cup	120	11%	1.5	0.5	15
Savory pot roast, 1 cup	120	11%	1.5	1	15
Savory vegetable, 1 cup	110	8%	1	0.5	18
Split pea & ham, 1 cup	170	13%	2.5	1	23

Product and Portion Size	Calories	% Cal from Fat	Total Fat (g)	Bad Fat (g)	Net Carbs (g)
Steak & potato, 1 cup	130	14%	2	0.5	16
Tomato cheese ravioli w/vegetables, 1 cup	160	17%	3	2	24
Turkey pot pie, 1 cup	180	35%	7	2	16
Campbell's Chunky Microwaveable					
Beef w/country vegetables, 1 cup	150	18%	3	1.5	16
Chicken & dumplings, 1 cup	190	43%	9	2	15
New England clam chowder, 1 cup	200	54%	12	2.5	15
Sirloin burger w/country vegetables, 1 cup	160	23%	4	2	14
Campbell's Healthy Choice					
Bean & ham, 1 cup	170	12%	2.5	1	23
Chunky beef & potato, 1 cup	110	9%	1	0	17
Fiesta chicken, 1 cup	100	15%	2	0.5	14
Garden vegetable , 1 cup	120	8%	1	0	21
New England clam chowder, 1 cup	110	9%	1.5	1	18
Roasted chicken w/garlic, 1 cup	120	13%	2	0	19
Split pea & ham, 1 cup	170	12%	2.5	1	26
Vegetable beef, 1 cup	130	8%	1	0	20
Zesty gumbo, 1 cup	100	20%	2	1	13

Product and Portion Size	Calories	% Cal from Fat	Total Fat (g)	Bad Fat (g)	Net Carbs (g)
Campbell's Healthy Request					
Chicken noodle, ½ cup	60	30%	2	0.5	7
Cream of celery, ½ cup	70	26%	2	0.5	11
Cream of mushroom, ½ cup	70	26%	2	0.5	9
Minestrone, ½ cup	80	6%	0.5	0	12
Vegetable beef, ½ cup	90	10%	1	0.5	12
Campbell's Select					
Beef w/roasted barley, 1 cup	130	7%	1	0.5	20
Chicken vegetable medley, 1 cup	110	4%	0.5	0.5	17
Creamy chicken alfredo, 1 cup	180	35%	7	1	16
Fiesta vegetable, 1 cup	120	38%	0.5	0	20
Italian style wedding, 1 cup	110	20%	2.5	2	14
Minestrone, 1 cup	100	5%	0.5	0	17
New England clam chowder, 98% fat free, 1 cup	110	12%	1.5	0	14
Potato broccoli cheese, 1 cup	120	30%	4	1	14
Roasted beef tips, 1 cup	120	11%	1.5	0.5	15
Roasted chicken w/rotini, 1 cup	100	5%	0.5	0.5	14
Savory lentil, 1 cup	140	3%	0.5	0.5	21

Product and Portion Size	Calories	% Cal from Fat	Total Fat (g)	Bad Fat (g)	Net Carbs (g)
Split pea w/roasted ham, 1 cup	160	6%	1	0	24
Tomato garden, 1 cup	100	5%	0.5	0.5	19
Vegetable medley, 1 cup	100	5%	0.5	0	18
Campbell's Soup at Hand					
Blended vegetable medley, 1 container	100	14%	1.5	0.5	15
Chicken & stars, 1 container	60	23%	1.5	0.5	8
Cream of broccoli, 1 container	150	42%	7	2	10
Mexican style fiesta, 1 container	150	30%	5	2.5	18
Pizza, 1 container	140	6%	1	0.5	25
Velvety potato, 1 container	160	39%	7	1	17
Imagine					
Crab bisque, 8 oz	130	35%	5	3	16
Lobster bisque, 1 cup	130	35%	5	3	15
Organic creamy broccoli, 1 cup	60	25%	1.5	0	8
Organic creamy butternut squash, 1 cup	90	17%	2	0	16
Organic creamy chicken, 1 cup	70	21%	1.5	0	11
Organic creamy sweet corn, 1 cup	120	20%	3	0.6	17
Organic creamy sweet potato, 1 cup	110	9%	1.5	0	22
Organic creamy tomato basil, 1 cup	90	17%	1.5	0	15

Product and Portion Size	Calories	% Cal from Fat	Total Fat (g)	Bad Fat (g)	Net Carbs (g)
Lipton Cup of Soup					
Asian beef noodle, 1 envelope	70	14%	1	0	14
Broccoli cheese, 1 envelope	90	17%	1.5	1	17
Chicken noodle, 1 envelope	80	6%	0.5	0	17
Cream of chicken, 1 envelope	70	21%	1.5	0	14
Spring vegetable, 1 envelope	50	0%	0	0	10
Tomato w/croutons, 1 envelope	90	28%	2.5	0	17
Progresso—50% less sodium					
Chicken gumbo, 1 cup	110	13%	1.5	0.5	16
Chicken noodle, 1 cup	90	17%	1.5	0	11
Garden vegetable, 1 cup	100	0%	0	0	19
Minestrone, 1 cup	120	13%	2	0.5	20
Progresso—Rich & Hearty					
Beef barley vegetable, 1 cup	130	8%	1	0.5	19
Chicken corn chowder, 1 cup	210	43%	9	2.5	21
Chicken & homestyle noodles, 1 cup	110	18%	2	0.5	13
Chicken pot pie style, 1 cup	170	29%	6	1.5	19
New England clam chowder, 1 cup	190	42%	9	2	20

Product and Portion Size	Calories	% Cal from Fat	Total Fat (g)	Bad Fat (g)	Net Carbs (g)
Sirloin steak & vegetables, 1 cup	130	15%	2	1	19
Steak & homestyle noodles, 1 cup	120	21%	3	1	15
Steak & sautéed mushrooms, 1 cup	110	14%	2	0.5	17
Progresso—Traditional					
Beef & baked potato, 1 cup	100	20%	2.5	1	14
Beef barley, 1 cup	140	25%	2.5	0.5	13
Beef barley, 98% f-f, 1 cup	120	13%	1.5	0.5	16
Beef & mushroom, 1 cup	100	5%	0.5	0	12
Beef & vegetables, 1 cup	100	5%	1	0	15
Chickaria, 1 cup	130	35%	5	1.5	11
Chicken & barley, 1 cup	100	25%	2.5	0.5	13
Chicken cheese enchilada, Carb Monitor, 1 cup	170	65%	12	4	7
Chicken noodle, 1 cup	100	20%	2.5	0.5	13
Chicken noodle, 99% f-f, 1 cup	100	15%	2	0.5	11
Chicken & rotini, 1 cup	100	20%	2	0.5	12
Chicken sausage gumbo, 1 cup	130	27%	4	1.5	17
Chicken vegetable, Carb monitor, 1 cup	70	21%	2	1	6
Chicken & wild rice, 1 cup	100	15%	1.5	0.5	14

Product and Portion Size	Calories	% Cal from Fat	Total Fat (g)	Bad Fat (g)	Net Carbs (g)
Homestyle chicken, 1 cup	100	15%	2	0	13
Italian style wedding, 1 cup	130	35%	5	2	14
New England clam chowder, 1 cup	190	47%	10	2.5	18
New England clam chowder, 99% f-f, 1 cup	120	17%	2	0	19
Split pea w/ham, 1 cup	150	17%	1	0.5	21
Turkey noodle, 1 cup	80	19%	1.5	0	11
Tuscan meatball, Carb Monitor, 1 cup	100	45%	5	2.5	8
Progresso—Vegetable Classics					
Creamy mushroom, 1 cup	130	69%	10	3	8
French onion, 1 cup	50	20%	1.5	0.5	7
Garden vegetable, 1 cup	90	0%	0	0	17
Lentil, 1 cup	150	13%	2	0.5	23
Minestrone, 1 cup	110	14%	2	0.5	15
Tomato basil, 1 cup	160	19%	3	0.5	29
Vegetable, 1 cup	80	6%	0.5	0	14
Vegetable Italiano, 1 cup	100	20%	2	0.5	15
Vegetarian vegetable w/barley, 1 cup	100	5%	0.5	0	16

Product and Portion Size	Calories	% Cal from Fat	Total Fat (g)	Bad Fat (g)	Net Carbs (g)
Top Ramen					
Beef, ½ pkg	190	32%	7	3.5	25
Cajun chicken, ½ pkg	180	33%	7	3.5	25
Chicken, ½ pkg	190	32%	7	3.5	24
Chicken Vegetable	190	37%	7	4	25
Oriental, ½ pkg	190	32%	7	3.5	25
Shrimp, ½ pkg	190	32%	7	3.5	25
Westbrae Natural					
Alabama black bean gumbo, 1 cup	140	0%	0	0	20
Hearty Milano minestrone, 1 cup	120	0%	0	0	18
Mediterranean lentil, 1 cup	140	0%	0	0	14
Old world split pea, 1 cup	150	0%	0	0	22
Santa Fe vegetable, 1 cup	160	0%	0	0	23
Tuscany tomato, ¾ cup	70	0%	0	0	16
SOUR CREAM					
Breakstone					
All natural, 2 Tbs	60	83%	5	3.5	1
Fat free, 2 Tbs	30	0%	0	0	5
Reduced fat, 2 Tbs	40	75%	3	2	2

Product and Portion Size	Calories	% Cal from Fat	Total Fat (g)	Bad Fat (g)	Net Carbs (g)
Daisy					
Light, 2 Tbs	40	63%	2.5	2	2
No fat, 2 Tbs	20	0%	0	0	1
Regular, 2 Tbs	60	75%	5	3.5	1
Knudsen					
Fat-free, 2 Tbs	30	0%	0	0	5
Hampshire, 2 Tbs	60	83%	6	3.5	1
Light, 2 Tbs	30	50%	2	1	2
SOY BEVERAGES					
Edensoy					
Carob, organic, 8 oz	170	21%	4	0.5	27
Chocolate, organic, 8 oz	180	17%	4	1	27
Extra original, 8 oz	130	27%	4	0.5	12
Extra vanilla, 8 oz	150	17%	3	0	22
Light, original, 8 oz	100	20%	2	0	15
Light, vanilla, 8 oz	110	9%	1	0	22
Original, 8 oz	140	29%	5	0.5	13
Vanilla, 8 oz	150	17%	3	0.5	23

Product and Portion Size	Calories	% Cal from Fat	Total Fat (g)	Bad Fat (g)	Net Carbs (g)
Pacific					
Organic soy, plain, low fat, 8 oz	70	29%	2.5	0	8
Organic soy, vanilla, low fat, 8 oz	80	25%	2.5	0	8
Organic soy, ultra, plain, 8 oz	120	29%	4	0.5	11
Organic soy, ultra, vanilla, 8 oz	130	27%	4	0.5	13
Silk					
Chai, 8 oz	130	23%	3.5	0.5	19
Chocolate, 8 oz	140	21%	3.5	0.5	21
Enhanced, 8 oz	110	41%	5	0.5	7
Light chocolate, 8 oz	120	13%	1.5	0	20
Light vanilla, 8 oz	80	25%	2	0	9
Mocha, 8 oz	140	21%	3.5	0.5	22
Plain, 8 oz	100	35%	4	0.5	7
Silk Live! Blueberry, 1 container	230	15%	4	0.5	39
Silk Live! Mango, 1 container	230	15%	4	0.5	38
Silk Live! Peach, 1 container	220	16%	4	0.5	35
Silk Live! Strawberry, 1 container	220	16%	4	0.5	37
Vanilla, 8 oz	100	30%	3.5	0.5	9

Product and Portion Size	Calories	% Cal from Fat	Total Fat (g)	Bad Fat (g)	Net Carbs (g)
Very vanilla, 8 oz	130	27%	4	0.5	18
SOY SAUCE—See "Sauces"					
SOYBEANS (also see "Tofu")					
Cascadian Farm, edamame, ⅔ cup	**120**	**42%**	**5**	**0.5**	**6**
Fresh, cooked, no salt, 1 cup	**298**	**43%**	**15**	**2**	**7**
Roasted, no salt, 1 oz	**133**	**45%**	**7**	**1**	**4**
SOY SNACKS					
Hain, caramel, 7 pcs	40	0%	0	0	7
Hain, ranch, 9 pcs	60	33%	2	0	7
Hain, white cheddar munchies, 9 pcs	60	42%	2.5	0.5	5
SPAGHETTI—See "Pasta"					
SPAGHETTI SQUASH, cooked, no salt, 1 cup	42	8%	0	0	8
SPINACH					
Fresh, cooked, drained, 1 cup	**41**	**9%**	**0**	**0**	**3**
Fresh, raw, 1 cup	**7**	**14%**	**0**	**0**	**0**
Birds Eye, chopped or leaf, frozen, ⅓ cup	**30**	**0%**	**0**	**0**	**2**
Birds Eye, creamed w/real cream, ½ cup	**100**	**63%**	**7**	**3**	**6**
Green Giant, frozen, no sauce, ½ cup	**25**	**0%**	**0**	**0**	**2**

Product and Portion Size	Calories	% Cal from Fat	Total Fat (g)	Bad Fat (g)	Net Carbs (g)
Green Giant, frozen, creamed, ½ cup	**70**	**36%**	**2.5**	**1.5**	**8**
Green Giant, frozen, cut leaf /butter, ½ cup	**30**	**33%**	**1**	**0**	**2**
S&W, canned, leaf, ½ cup	**30**	**0%**	**0**	**0**	**2**
SQUASH. See specific types					
STRAWBERRIES, fresh raw, 1 cup	49	8%	0	0	9
Cascadian farm, frozen, 1 cup	45	0%	0	0	10
STUFFING					
Pepperidge Farm					
Corn bread, ¾ cup	170	11%	2	0	31
Country style, ¾ cup	140	6%	1	0	25
Cube, ¾ cup	140	6%	1	0	26
One step chicken, ½ cup	160	23%	4	1	23
One step turkey, ½ cup	170	37%	7	1	22
Sage & onion, ¾ cup	140	6%	1	0	23
Stove Top					
Chicken, ⅙ box	110	9%	1	0	19
Chicken, lower sodium, ⅙ box	110	9%	1	0	20
Chicken w/whole wheat, ⅕ box	100	14%	1.5	0	15

Product and Portion Size	Calories	% Cal from Fat	Total Fat (g)	Bad Fat (g)	Net Carbs (g)
Cornbread one step, ⅛ box	120	25%	3	0	18
Homestyle herb one step, ⅛ box	110	23%	2.5	0	18
Pork, ⅙ box	110	8%	1	0	19
Turkey, ⅙ box	110	9%	1	0	19
SUGAR					
Brown, 1 tsp	11	0%	0	0	3
Powdered, 1 tsp	10	0%	0	0	2
White, granulated, 1 tsp	15	0%	0	0	4
SUNFLOWER SEEDS, dried, 1 oz	161	73%	14	1	2
Planters, dry roasted, 1 oz	180	72%	15	1.5	3
SWEET POTATOES					
Baked in skin w/salt, 1 medium	103	1%	0	0	20
Green Giant candied, frozen, ¾ cup	240	40%	7	2.5	38
Green Giant, sweet potato casserole, frozen, 1 cup	200	45%	10	3	25
McCain sweet potato fry, 3 oz	120	33%	3	0.5	20
SWORDFISH, cooked, dry heat, 3 oz	**132**	**30%**	**4**	**1**	**0**
TACO SHELLS					
Old El Paso, 3 shells	150	40%	7	4	19
Taco Bell, 3 shells	150	40%	6	1	20

Product and Portion Size	Calories	% Cal from Fat	Total Fat (g)	Bad Fat (g)	Net Carbs (g)
TANGERINE, raw, 1 cup	103	5%	1	0	22
Minute Maid orange tangerine juice, 8 oz	110	0%	0	0	27
Noble, tangerine juice, 8 oz	125	0%	0	0	30
POM, tangerine juice, 8 oz	140	0%	0	0	34
TEA					
Celestial Seasonings					
All herbal, dessert, holiday, black teas, 1 bag	0	0%	0	0	0
Cinnamon spice teahouse chai, 3 Tbs	110	0%	0	0	25
Sweet coconut thai chai, 3 Tbs	110	0%	0	0	25
Vanilla ginger chai, 3 Tbs	110	0%	0	0	25
Lipton					
Chailatta, original, 3 Tbs	120	17%	2	0	21
Chailatta, vanilla, 3 Tbs	120	17%	2	0	19
Hot tea, black or green, 1 bag	0	0%	0	0	0
Iced green tea w/citrus, 8 oz	80	0%	0	0	21
Iced tea mix, sweetened, lemon, 1⅓ Tbs	70	0%	0	0	18
Iced tea mix, sweetened, raspberry, 1½ Tbs	80	0%	0	0	19
Original iced tea, bottles, 8 oz	80	0%	0	0	21
White tea w/tangerine, bottles, 8 oz	60	0%	0	0	16

Product and Portion Size	Calories	% Cal from Fat	Total Fat (g)	Bad Fat (g)	Net Carbs (g)
TEMPEH					
Lightlife, organic flax, 4 oz	220	25%	9	1.5	0
Lightlife, organic garden veggie, 4 oz	200	45%	10	1.5	3
Lightlife organic, three grain, 4 oz	230	35%	9	1.5	13
Lightlife organic, wild rice, 4 oz	230	27%	7	1	10
TOFU					
Fresh Tofu Inc.					
Baked stuffed, 1 pc	**160**	**25%**	**4.5**	**0.5**	**8**
Organic baked, 2 oz	**90**	**56%**	**6**	**1**	**1**
Mori-Nu					
Chinese spice seasoned, 3 oz	**50**	**40%**	**2**	**0**	**3**
Enriched silken, firm, 3 oz	**70**	**36%**	**2.5**	**0**	**6**
Japanese miso seasoned, 3 oz	**60**	**42%**	**2.5**	**0**	**3**
Silken, extra firm, 3 oz	**48**	**31%**	**1.5**	**0**	**2**
Silken, lite extra firm, 3 oz	**35**	**14%**	**0.5**	**0**	**1**
Silken, soft, 3 oz	**45**	**44%**	**2.5**	**0**	**2**
Nasoya					
Chinese spice firm, ¼ pkg	**90**	**50%**	**5**	**1**	**2**
Extra firm, ⅕ pkg	**80**	**45%**	**4.5**	**0.5**	**2**

Product and Portion Size	Calories	% Cal from Fat	Total Fat (g)	Bad Fat (g)	Net Carbs (g)
Garlic & onion, ¼ pkg	**90**	**50%**	**5**	**1**	**2**
Lite firm, ¼ pkg	**40**	**34%**	**1.5**	**0**	**0**
Silken, ⅕ pkg	**45**	**40%**	**2**	**0**	**1**
Soft, ⅕ pkg	**60**	**45%**	**3**	**1**	**0**
TOMATOES					
Fresh, red, cooked, 1 cup	43	5%	0	0	8
Fresh, red cherry, 1 cup	31	13%	0	0	5
Fresh, red, 1 medium	26	13%	0	0	5
Fresh, red plum, 1	13	13%	0	0	2
Fresh, yellow, chopped, 1 cup	21	14%	0	0	3
Canned					
Del Monte, diced w/garlic & onion, ½ cup	40	15%	0.5	0	7
Del Monte, diced pasta style, ½ cup	45	0%	0	0	9
Del Monte, stewed, Mexican, ½ cup	35	0%	0	0	7
Del Monte, wedges, ½ cup	35	0%	0	0	7
Eden Organic, crushed w/basil, ¼ cup	20	0%	0	0	2
Eden Organic, diced w/green chilis, ½ cup	30	0%	0	0	3
Eden Organic, whole, ½ cup	30	0%	0	0	3

Product and Portion Size	Calories	% Cal from Fat	Total Fat (g)	Bad Fat (g)	Net Carbs (g)
Muir Glen, crushed w/basil, ¼ cup	25	0%	0	0	4
Muir Glen, diced w/Italian herbs, ½ cup	30	0%	0	0	5
Muir Glen, whole, fire roasted, ½ cup	25	0%	0	0	4
Muir Glen, whole, peeled plum, ½ cup	25	0%	0	0	4
Progresso, crushed, ¼ cup	20	0%	0	0	3
Progresso, diced, ½ cup	25	0%	0	0	4
Progresso, whole peeled w/basil, ½ cup	20	0%	0	0	3
TOMATO JUICE					
Campbell's, Healthy Request, 8 oz	50	0%	0	0	0
Campbell's, original, 8 oz	50	0%	0	0	0
Del Monte, 8 oz	50	0%	0	0	1
TOMATO PASTE/PUREE					
Hunt's, paste, 2 Tbs	25	0%	0	0	4
Hunt's, paste, no salt, 2 Tbs	30	0%	0	0	4
Hunt's, paste, w/basil, garlic, oregano, 2 Tbs	25	0%	0	0	4
Hunt's, puree, 4 oz	30	0%	0	0	5
Muir Glen, paste, 2 Tbs	30	0%	0	0	5
Muir Glen, puree, ¼ cup	25	0%	0	0	5

Product and Portion Size	Calories	% Cal from Fat	Total Fat (g)	Bad Fat (g)	Net Carbs (g)
S&W, paste, 2 Tbs	30	0%	0	0	5
S&W, puree, ¼ cup	30	0%	0	0	0
TOPPINGS, DESSERT					
Cool Whip, chocolate, 2 Tbs	25	100%	1.5	1.5	2
Cool Whip, French vanilla, 2 Tbs	25	100%	1.5	1.5	2
Cool Whip, lite, 2 Tbs	20	50%	1	1	3
Cool Whip, regular, 2 Tbs	25	60%	1.5	1.5	2
Cool Whip, sugar free, 2 Tbs	20	50%	1	1	3
Smucker's, butterscotch caramel, 2 Tbs	130	8%	1	0.5	29
Smucker's, Dove dark chocolate, 2 Tbs	140	32%	5	1.5	21
Smucker's, Plate Scrapers caramel, 2 Tbs	100	0%	0	0	25
Smucker's, Plate Scrapers raspberry, 2 Tbs	100	0%	0	0	25
Smucker's, Plate Scrapers vanilla, 2 Tbs	110	9%	1	0	24
Smucker's, special recipe hot fudge, 2 Tbs	140	29%	4	1	21
TUNA					
Chicken of the Sea					
Chunk, lite in oil, 2 oz	**110**	**45%**	**6**	**1**	**0**
Chunk lite in water, 2 oz	**60**	**8%**	**0.5**	**0**	**0**

Product and Portion Size	Calories	% Cal from Fat	Total Fat (g)	Bad Fat (g)	Net Carbs (g)
Chunk white in water, 2 oz	**60**	**17%**	**1**	**0**	**0**
Genova tonno in olive oil, 2 oz	**130**	**54%**	**8**	**1**	**0**
Premium, albacore, pouch, 2 oz	**60**	**17%**	**1**	**0**	**0**
Solid white albacore, in oil, 2 oz	**90**	**33%**	**3**	**1**	**0**
Solid white albacore in water, 2 oz	**70**	**14%**	**1**	**0**	**0**
Yellowfin solid light, water, 2 oz	**70**	**14%**	**1**	**0**	**0**
Starkist					
Chunk light pouch, 3 oz	**90**	**10%**	**1**	**0**	**0**
Chunk light water, can, 2 oz	**60**	**8%**	**0.5**	**0**	**0**
Gourmet choice fillet, water, 2 oz	**60**	**17%**	**1**	**0**	**0**
Solid white albacore, water, 2 oz	**70**	**14%**	**1**	**0**	**0**
TURKEY					
Dark meat, roasted, 1 oz	53	35%	2	1	0
Light meat, roasted, 1 oz	44	18%	1	0	0
Louis Rich, breast & white, 1 oz	28	18%	1	0	1
Louis Rich, pure ground, 4 oz	190	58%	12	3.5	0
Louis Rich, smoked white, 95% f-f, 1 oz	30	33%	1	0	1
TURNIP, cooked, no salt, 1 cup	34	3%	0	0	5

Product and Portion Size	Calories	% Cal from Fat	Total Fat (g)	Bad Fat (g)	Net Carbs (g)
VEAL					
Breast, boneless, lean, 3 oz	185	40%	8	3	0
Leg, lean, 3 oz	128	10%	3	1	0
Loin, lean, 3 oz	149	36%	6	2	0
Rib, lean, 3 oz	185	32%	7	2	0
Sirloin, lean, 3 oz	143	33%	5	2	0
VEGETABLE JUICE					
Knudsen, Very Veggie, low sodium, 8 oz	50	0%	0	0	9
Knudsen, Very Veggie, original, 8 oz	50	0%	0	0	9
Knudsen, Very Veggie, spicy, 8 oz	50	0%	0	0	9
V-8, calcium enriched, 8 oz	50	0%	0	0	9
V-8, low sodium, 8 oz	50	0%	0	0	8
V-8, picante, 8 oz	50	0%	0	0	8
V-8, 100%, 8 oz	50	0%	0	0	8
VEGETABLES, Mixed					
Canned					
Del Monte, homestyle medley, ½ cup	70	32%	2.5	0	9
Del Monte mixed, ½ cup	40	0%	0	0	6

Product and Portion Size	Calories	% Cal from Fat	Total Fat (g)	Bad Fat (g)	Net Carbs (g)
Del Monte mixed w/potatoes, ½ cup	45	0%	0	0	8
S&W mixed, ½ cup	45	0%	0	0	8
Birds Eye					
Asian in sesame ginger, 1 cup	60	15%	1	0	10
Baby corn & vegetable blend, ⅔ cup	50	18%	1	0	6
Baby pea & vegetable blend, ¾ cup	40	0%	0	0	5
Baby potato & vegetable blend, ¾ cup	40	0%	0	0	8
California blend & cheddar cheese, ½ cup	80	45%	4	2	7
Classic mixed, ⅔ cup	60	0%	0	0	10
Szechuan in sesame sauce, 1 cup	60	30%	2	0	7
Tuscan vegetables in herbed tomato, 1 cup	50	30%	2	0	5
Cascadian Farm					
California style blend, ⅔ cup	25	0%	0	0	3
Chinese stir fry, 1 cup	25	0%	0	0	4
Garden's blend, ¾ cup	50	0%	0	0	8
Thai stir fry, ¾ cup	25	0%	0	0	10
Green Giant					
Baby vegetable medley, ¾ cup	40	25%	1	0	7

Product and Portion Size	Calories	% Cal from Fat	Total Fat (g)	Bad Fat (g)	Net Carbs (g)
Boxed alfredo, ¾ cup	60	33%	2	1	7
Garden medley, ½ cup prep.	70	7%	0.5	0	12
Plain mixed, ½ cup prep.	50	0%	0	0	9
Simply steam garden medley, ½ cup prep.	50	10%	0.5	0	10
Szechuan vegetables, ¾ cup	50	10%	0.5	0	7
Teriyaki vegetables, 1¼ cup	70	57%	4.5	2	5
VINEGAR					
Eden Foods, apple cider or red wine organic, 1 Tbs	0	0%	0	0	0
Eden Foods, brown rice, organic, 1 Tbs	2	0%	0	0	0
Eden Foods, ume plum, imported, 1 tsp	0	0%	0	0	0
Progresso, balsamic, 1 Tbs	10	0%	0	0	2
WAFFLES—See Frozen Breakfast; Pancake/Waffle					
WALNUTS, black, dried, 1 oz	**175**	**80%**	**17**	**1**	**1**
Planters, walnuts, 1 oz	**210**	**86%**	**20**	**2**	**4**
WATERMELON, 1 cup balls	46	4%	0	0	11
WHITEFISH, cooked, 3 oz	146	39%	6	1	0
Smoked, 3 oz	92	8%	1	0	0
WINE, red table (average values), 5 oz	125	0%	0	0	4

Product and Portion Size	Calories	% Cal from Fat	Total Fat (g)	Bad Fat (g)	Net Carbs (g)
Rose table (average values), 3 oz	73	0%	0	0	1
White table (average values), 5 oz	122	0%	0	0	4
YAM, boiled or baked, no salt, cubes, 1 cup	158	1%	0	0	33
Canned, candied (S&W), ½ cup	170	0%	0	0	42
YOGURT					
Columbo					
Classic banana strawberry, 8 oz	230	9%	2	1.5	47
Classic blueberry, cherry, peach, raspberry, strawberry, 8 oz	220	9%	2	1.5	42
Classic vanilla, 8 oz	190	13%	2.5	1.5	33
Light: blueberry, cherry vanilla, keylime, mixed berry, peach, raspberry, strawberry, 8 oz	120	0%	0	0	21
Low fat, plain, 8 oz	100	0%	0	0	16
Low fat, strawberry or vanilla, 8 oz	220	9%	2.5	1.5	42
Dannon					
Activia, prune, 4 oz	110	18%	2	1	19
Activia, strawberry, 4 oz	110	18%	2	1	19
Activia, vanilla, 4 oz	110	18%	2	1.5	19

Product and Portion Size	Calories	% Cal from Fat	Total Fat (g)	Bad Fat (g)	Net Carbs (g)
DanActive, blueberry, cranberry/raspberry, strawberry, or vanilla, 3.3 oz	90	17%	1.5	1	17
DanActive, plain, 3.3 oz	90	22%	1.5	1.5	15
Fruit on Bottom, apple cinnamon, 6 oz	150	10%	1.5	1	27
Fruit on Bottom, cherry, 6 oz	140	11%	1.5	1	26
Fruit on Bottom, mixed berry, 6 oz	150	10%	1.5	1.5	26
Fruit on Bottom, pineapple, 6 oz	150	10%	1.5	1.5	26
Frusion, cherry berry blend, 10 oz	260	12%	3.5	2	49
Frusion, pina colada, 10 oz	260	12%	3.5	2	50
Frusion, strawberry blend, 10 oz	260	12%	3.5	2	50
La Crème, all flavors, 4 oz	140	32%	5	3	19
Stonyfield					
Cultured O'Soy, blueberry, 6 oz	170	12%	2	0	29
Cultured O'Soy, chocolate, 6 oz	160	16%	3	0	24
Cultured O'Soy, vanilla, 6 oz	150	13%	2	0	22
Fat-free, apricot mango, 6 oz	130	0%	0	0	24
Fat-free, chocolate underground, 6 oz	170	0%	0	0	34
Fat-free, French vanilla, 8 oz	180	0%	0	0	33

Product and Portion Size	Calories	% Cal from Fat	Total Fat (g)	Bad Fat (g)	Net Carbs (g)
Fat-free, lotsa lemon, 6 oz	140	0%	0	0	26
Fat-free, peach, 6 oz	120	0%	0	0	23
Fat-free, plain, 8 oz	100	0%	0	0	15
Light, all flavors, 6 oz	100	0%	0	0	25
Smoothies, reg., banana berry, 10 oz	250	10%	3	2	43
Smoothies, reg., peach, 10 oz	250	10%	3	2	45
Smoothies, reg., strawberry or vanilla, 10 oz	250	10%	3	2	42
Smoothies, light, banana berry, 10 oz	130	0%	0	0	38
Smoothies, light, peach, 10 oz	130	0%	0	0	38
Smoothies, light, strawberry, 10 oz	130	0%	0	0	38
Yoplait					
Go-Gurt, smoothies, all flavors, 1 bottle	120	4%	0.5	0	23
Grande, all flavors, 8 oz	220	9%	2.5	1.5	42
Grande, plain, 8 oz	130	0%	0	0	19
Light, all flavors, 6 oz	100	0%	0	0	19
Nouriche, all flavors, 1 container	260	0%	0	0	50
Original, most flavors, 6 oz	170	9%	1.5	1	33
Original, coconut cream, 6 oz	190	13%	3	2	34

Product and Portion Size	Calories	% Cal from Fat	Total Fat (g)	Bad Fat (g)	Net Carbs (g)
Original, pina colada, 6 oz	170	9%	2	1.5	33
Original, plain, 6 oz	100	0%	0	0	14
Smoothie, light, all flavors, 8 oz	90	0%	0	0	16
Smoothie, all flavors, 8 oz	190	11%	2.5	1.5	38
Thick & creamy, all flavors, 6 oz	190	16%	3.5	2	32
Whips! All chocolate flavors, 4 oz	160	22%	4	2.5	26
Whips! All other flavors, 4 oz	140	14%	2.5	2	25
YOGURT—Frozen					
Ben & Jerry's					
Cherry Garcia, low fat, ½ cup	170	15%	3	2	31
Chocolate fudge brownie, low fat, ½ cup	190	13%	2.5	1.5	34
Half baked, low fat, ½ cup	190	13%	3	1.5	34
Phish food, ½ cup	220	20%	4.5	3.5	40
Haagen-Dazs					
Chocolate fudge brownie, ½ cup	200	12%	2.5	1.5	33
Coffee, ½ cup	200	20%	4.5	2.5	31
Strawberry, f-f, ½ cup	140	0%	0	0	31
Vanilla, low fat, ½ cup	200	20%	4.5	2.5	31
Vanilla raspberry swirl, ½ cup	170	15%	2.5	1.5	32

Product and Portion Size	Calories	% Cal from Fat	Total Fat (g)	Bad Fat (g)	Net Carbs (g)
Stonyfield					
After dark chocolate, organic, nonfat, ½ cup	100	0%	0	0	20
Cookies 'n cream, low fat, ½ cup	130	7%	1	0	25
Gotta have vanilla, organic, nonfat, ½ cup	100	0%	0	0	21
Javalanche, organic, nonfat, ½ cup	100	0%	0	0	21
Minty chocolate chip, low fat, ½ cup	170	19%	3	1.5	24
ZUCCHINI, cooked, no salt, 1 cup	29	3%	0	0	4
Raw, w/skin, 1 cup	20	9%	0	0	3
Canned, w/tomato (Del Monte), ½ cup	30	0%	0	0	6

NEED SOMETHING NEW TO READ?

Download it Now!

Visit www.harpercollinsebooks.com
to choose from thousands of titles
you can easily download to your
computer or PDA.

Save 20% off the printed book price.
Ordering is easy and secure.

HarperCollins e-books

Download to your laptop, PDA, or phone for convenient, immediate, or on-the-go reading. Visit www.harpercollinsebooks.com or other online e-book retailers.

Visit www.AuthorTracker.com for exclusive information on your favorite HarperCollins authors.

Available wherever books are sold or please call 1-800-331-3761 to order.

HRE 0307